Praise for
THE BIG M

"*The Big M* feels like a heartfelt conversation with a trusted friend. It reminds us that we are not alone. By sharing our stories, we can reshape the menopause experience together. With warmth and wisdom, this book leaves you feeling informed, empowered, and more connected to yourself and others on the journey."

—Nedra Glover Tawwab, *New York Times* bestselling author of *Set Boundaries, Find Peace* and *Drama Free*

"As varied in experience as it is refreshingly and (yes) brutally honest, *The Big M* offers a chorus of voices to enlighten, guide, and buoy any woman through the joys, the trials, and the ultimate awakening/redefining that occurs in midlife."

—Cathi Hanauer, editor of *New York Times* bestseller *The Bitch in the House*

"At last, a corrective breaking the pervasive silence around menopause and its many effects on the body and mind, effects that have previously blindsided one uninformed generation after another. *The Big M* gathers some of the most compelling writers of our time, voicing a wide array of menopause experiences, and revealing ways in which—counter to gendered ageism's messaging—we gain empowerment in our crone years."

—Sari Botton, founder of *Oldster Magazine*, and author of *And You May Find Yourself…*

the BIG M

13 WRITERS TAKE BACK
THE STORY OF MENOPAUSE

edited by

LIDIA YUKNAVITCH

GCP

GRAND
CENTRAL

New York   Boston

Grand Central Publishing
Hachette Book Group
1290 Avenue of the Americas, New York, NY 10104
grandcentralpublishing.com
@grandcentralpub

First Trade Paperback Edition: January 2026

Grand Central Publishing is a division of Hachette Book Group, Inc. The Grand Central Publishing name and logo is a registered trademark of Hachette Book Group, Inc.

The publisher is not responsible for websites (or their content) that are not owned by the publisher.

The Hachette Speakers Bureau provides a wide range of authors for speaking events. To find out more, go to hachettespeakersbureau.com or email HachetteSpeakers@hbgusa.com.

Grand Central Publishing books may be purchased in bulk for business, educational, or promotional use. For information, please contact your local bookseller or the Hachette Book Group Special Markets Department at special.markets@hbgusa.com.

Print book interior design by Taylor Navis.

Library of Congress Cataloging-in-Publication Data has been applied for.

ISBNs: 9781538765548 (trade paperback edition), 9781538765562 (ebook), 9781538783092 (large print)

Printed in the United States of America

LSC-C

Printing 1, 2025

CONTENTS

CONTENTS

FOREWORD

By Dr. Jen Gunter

Menopause is a universally shared experience among those of us born with ovaries. It is normal; a physiologic process, much like puberty in reverse. Yet, for generations it has been shrouded in silence, stigmatized by societal taboos born from the patriarchy, as if a woman's currency begins and ends with fertility.

Thus the range of physical and emotional experiences that may accompany menopause are a mystery. How are we to know? It is rarely discussed, whether in the office with a health care professional, at home with a mother or sister or aunt, or even among friends. Our society has pathologized menopause as something so awful that it is best met with silence, even in our own thoughts!

As a result, we are bereft. Where are stories of menopause and beyond? The stories we tell—to ourselves and others—matter.

They help us understand ourselves and the world, influence our beliefs and expectations, pierce the illusion that we are each alone.

Am I normal? What do other women experience? When should I get help? How can you know when there is a menopausal shroud? The patriarchy has distorted the narrative for so long, controlling not just our bodies but our very own thoughts about them. But here, in these pages, an amazing collective of women says, "No more."

With fierce honesty, the essays within these pages confront the physical realities of the body and illuminate the emotional shifts and life experiences that may accompany menopause. These are stories of change. The writers give voice to the unspoken—blood, tampons, desire, dryness, endometriosis, fibroids, cancer, hot flashes, brain fog, and domestic violence. Some experiences directly related to menopause, and others a coincidence of timing. But there is also love, longing, and laughter. And contentment.

Some stories may offer an uncanny reflection of your own life, and others will be foreign, but both the affirmation of the known and the exploration of the unknown leave us stronger and better for the journey. This is the rich tapestry of women's lives.

Menopause is not just a phase of the body's life cycle but also a rite of passage deserving of stories. These writers graciously show us that there is a richness of women's experiences to be explored that does not stop with the last menstrual period. Here, we unearth joy, grief, transformation, and the importance of embracing our bodies in all seasons. There are moments of vulnerability as well as acts of defiance and reclamation. This is more than an account of biology; it is a testament to the resilience and strength of women who have navigated their bodies in a world that has often sought to minimize or silence their experiences. There is solidarity and a reminder of the importance of being seen, heard, and understood. This is a long overdue reckoning.

I wished I had read this in book form and not as an electronic document (as is typically required when you are asked to write something prepublication) because there were times I wanted to hold it to my chest.

What a joy to read such gifted writers who are not just breaking the silence of menopause but reclaiming the narrative. It is powerful medicine indeed.

INTRODUCTION

By Lidia Yuknavitch

THIS BLOOD IS MINE AGAIN

Make no mistake: We are here to unapologetically share our Big M stories.

We are reclaiming and naming our Big M stories in the face of prior stigmatizations and shame holes. We hereby break all the dams and restore the stories. Some of the stories will make you laugh, or cry, or hold your breath. Some of them you've never heard before, others will have you nodding your head *yes, yes, please keep saying that out loud.* Some stories will cull histories, cross cultures; others will chart a path. You may sometimes feel counted, or curious, or compassionate. Some will illuminate bold new possibilities and change our way of thinking about our own bodies and life choices. One thing all the stories and storytellers have in common: We are here to show you how many ways there are through. We are here to remind you that you are not alone.

Stories are meaning-making tools. What we tell each other matters because what we tell each other affects how we see our lives and how we live them. We are sharing the stories we wish someone had shared with us in the hopes that you can carry something with you on your own journeys. Advice, wisdom, good questions, shared fears, inspiration, camaraderie, solace, imagination. We are here to lock arms and say embodied story-telling matters. Our bodies carry everything that has ever happened to us, and thus history, the present tense, and the future carry traces of all of us too.

This blood is mine again is a kind of rallying cry. The declaration is meant to conjure a reclamation story. So many humans who bleed their way through life enter the space of giver, whether that means bearing and raising children, or entering caretaker roles or support stations, or inhabiting a feminized space we have traditionally called "woman." We'd like to turn back on that word "woman," have a look. Part of the challenge is to both honor our past understandings of the word "woman" (so many humans whose bones we are standing on), as well as imagine the word, the identity, the space of being a fully human person moving through this stage of their life as opening, unfurling, extending into more expansive meanings and possibilities.

Reclaiming our own blood as we enter the time and space where we do not bleed out into the world is not just about that red, vital fluid, or any biologic essentialism. Reclaiming our blood can mean letting former biologic meanings that felt restricting become more fluid and playful. Reclaiming our blood can also mean standing up inside our own lineages, recognizing and honoring ancestors, resisting previous oppressions and repressions, laying down the bodies of ghosts we no longer need to carry, imagining new meanings for body, self, family, home, origin, roots, kinship, love. In short, reclaiming our blood is a form of restorying.

Tens of thousands of people a day around the globe step into menopause. In the United States alone, more than six thousand each day. Menopause is an embodied experience to be sure, but we suggest to you that it is also a real place, a threshold. We step into it. We cross over. We inhabit. We occupy. And as any person who has ever entered this place knows, the runway, the lead-up to menopause, can last anywhere from two to fifteen years (average: four to five). As Hope Reese noted in her 2023 article in the *New York Times*, "While hot flashes are a well-known hallmark, perimenopause can cause dozens of other symptoms including brain fog, sore breasts, poor sleeping and anxiety."[*] That list doesn't even begin to cover the hundreds of other symptoms people who experience perimenopause and menopause share with each other. Let's eyeball a bigger list. It will be okay. We are looking at it together. The list isn't going to kill us just from reading it:

Weight gain, gut and digestion hijinks, mood roller coasters, irregular bleeding, odd blood-floods, weird sex drive fluctuations (in all directions!), dryness, itch and ache up in the nethers

---

[*] Hope Reese, "7 Books to Guide You Through Menopause," *New York Times*, July 18, 2023, https://www.nytimes.com/2023/07/18/well/live/menopause-books.html.

(they call this vaginal atrophy, which is the worst name in the history of ever, so I've renamed it vaginal revolution—but seriously, I thought I had a cactus growing all up in there), headaches, fatigue, joint pain, odd tingles in your hands or feet, the bloats, digestive tricks, memory loss or just the inability to remember what memory even *is* any longer, thinning hair, brittle nails, dizziness and even fainting, jackknifing heartbeat, changes in body smells, changes in pee (all the time, not enough), sometimes an increase in UTIs (this happened to me rather dramatically), thinning uterus, rearrangement of internal organs (dropping—don't panic. It's a thing), and of course depression—especially if someone is experiencing one or all of these altered states and has no one to share them with.

Take a breath.

Take another breath.

Now take a hot bath, or a cold plunge, or go on a long walk, or swim, or forest bathe, or go cook something, write something, paint something, collect something—rocks, feathers, beads—cuddle with your dog or cat, watch birds, watch light or water move, meditate, exercise, talk to ghosts, get a massage, watch a movie that makes you laugh your ass off, or cry your face off, hit the heavy bag, climb a rock wall or mountain, eat chocolate and drink wine—do *something* you know gives you solace. We do know what to give ourselves, we just don't do it sometimes.

This time, you are not alone.

Take our stories with you. No, really. Carry the book around with you when you feel like things are difficult. Put it under your pillow and offer no explanation, or say, I'm busy dreaming of changing the world. Take our histories, our blood, our sweat, our tears, take our laughter as medicine, take our good imaginations.

For everything on that list and all the states of being not on that list, there are hundreds of story paths available to you. We just have to find them together and step into them.

In addition to a reclamation story, by collecting our different experiences this book shows you the stories behind the word "symptoms." We want to demystify and de-pathologize menopause. We want to testify. I know so many menopausal people who went into their doctor's offices believing they were going nuts or seriously ill, desperately bleating, What's wrong with me? And I hear about so many of them being told something like, oh, here's a long list of what is wrong with you, or whoa, this is all in your head, or, well, yes, this is how it is, nothing to be done. Like the goal is to fit our varied experiences into a prefabricated list, or fit us all into a monostory of inevitable duress.

Then there are the people who told their spouses or partners about what it feels like in an actual body, daily, weekly, monthly, *for years*, and were met with disbelief, or judgment, or some form of shaming. This is a no-shame zone, though we speak our shame stories as a means of alchemy.

Even when people entering menopause tell their story to other people who are seemingly sympathetic, there can be a weird disconnect. Those too young to have arrived yet sometimes turn away or cringe, or their eyes just glaze over a bit. I mean, it can sound scary, which can leave the person trying to share the story feeling monstrous or icky about aging. Those whose embodied experiences are not shared by their own friends or family can feel outcast or ostracized, like *dang, that's not happening to ME, how can it be happening to YOU?* One of my closest friends, an incredibly smart, successful, loving, and creative person with access to all kinds of resources, said to me, "But it's just basically hot flashes and mood swings, right? Maybe insomnia? That's all I have." After I'd told her I thought I might be dying.

My own sister, bless her, had this to offer when I got there: "I barely noticed. It was easy." I couldn't be happier for her! But what do I do with that? My mother? Not. A. Word. Thank the cosmos for the matrilineal lines who preserve stories and hand something useful down. Without them we'd be fucked. Most of what I've learned has come from my *other* family, writers and artists who, when asked, throw it down for me.

Nothing is wrong with you. You are entering the next part of your life, through your body, and that is incredible but also complex, and we want to welcome you, cheer you on, fashion you a crown, bake you a cake, sit and cry with you when you need it, hold your hand when you are scared, kick down any doors that shut in front of you, go shopping, radically change your hair, go night swimming, arrive naked at the grocery store in herds, chain ourselves to fences in front of the White House, laugh our asses off, eat a bag of potato chips, peel out in a neon convertible singing at the top of our lungs with you on some road trip to nowhere, but always remind you, you are a goddamn secular miracle. Individually we are mighty, to be sure.

Together we mighty miracles are legion, and we can change the story for each other and for those on their way.

We are not the story they made of us.

All of us, at one time or another, could benefit from exploring resources from experts in gynecology, endocrinology, and other important fields orbiting our entrances into menopause; this book inhabits storytelling space and embodied experiences. Maybe even like stepping into your erotic power story, whatever that means to you.

Several of the stories in this collection begin with first blood, otherwise known as having your first period. I thought about that narrative a lot—about puberty being an origin story for a blood life cycle, and that this blood life cycle is one way of telling the story of a life. You know, rather than "my first kiss" or "the first sex I ever had" (neither of which were meaningful to me personally, by the way, not like "my first movie viewing experience" or "my first book that felt like it happened to me"). Marking their first period as a point of origin lets someone talk about their life differently than some other origin point. Cheryl Strayed's essay reflects on the strength available even inside moments where we were made to feel shame, and will have readers remembering their own early blood-born moments with the possibility of wonder and awe. Joey Soloway's blood-flood essay will make you laugh out loud, and as we all know, laughter is sometimes powerful—even radical medicine.

In addition to reclamation, these stories are global, intersectional, and they inhabit more than one kind of embodiment, reminding us that no single story is universal in the ways we've been trained to pretend. The very differences between our bodies and lived experiences are what collect us into chorus. Menopause has no country of origin but the body. Nguyễn Phan Quế Mai's essay travels the strata beginning with growing up in rural Việt Nam in the '70s and '80s and into what it feels like in the present tense of being a Vietnamese woman. Julia Alvarez brings us through generations to the other side of menopause with joy and wisdom. Lan Samantha Chang weaves her way through generational understandings and changes in how Chinese immigrants face off with the past and the present, how people carry generational stories in their own bodies.

Some of the essays pull in threads from the world around us sociologically. Monica Drake's essay explores single motherhood, divorce law, and the devaluing of wives and mothers underlying the body changes that mark lives. Gina Frangello's essay stages what happens at the zenith of freedom and midlife sexuality as they crash into difficult medical diagnoses, personal and familial. Nana-Ama Danquah's deep dive into a history of her uterus speaks eloquently to difficult territories of depression, trauma, and the battering messages women receive about their reproductive anatomy, arriving finally at a place of reinvention and peace. Roxane Gay's essay reminds us that the body is a world we inhabit on our own terms, one with its own ever-emerging story, a story that can change at any moment in our lives.

And more than one essay asks us to de-center the human as we reach for our next forms. Pam Houston's essay delights and inspires through the relationship she found with Icelandic ponies and her beloved dogs. Darcey Steinke's essay moves from the personal through our animal ancestors to reveal how death and decay stories give way to their counterpoints, desire, fecundity, creativity. Reyna Grande brings us through the imagery of gardening and animal life to refocus the story of menopause on growth, even as difficulty may mark some stages. There are fables and folktales where living creatures real and imagined remind us that shape-shifting is beautiful.

It is as if we need many bodies—and thus many stories—to open up the story of menopause, rather than one body that is endlessly pathologized by societies that want to keep our stories small and quiet. These stories are not small and quiet.

To gently usher us into these stories, consider the phrase "this blood is mine again" as a portal. Many readers have likely heard of The Grandmother hypothesis. Menopause only exists in certain species, such as primates and whales and Asian elephants, to name a few. Anthropologists hypothesize that menopause can be understood as an evolutionary trait—by ceasing to reproduce, these mighty matriarchs are likely to live longer, and be prized by their communities for the contributions they can make benefiting the collective. Their value is not sidelined or invisible. Their value to the group is vital to the existence of the community. Those of us still standing are not dead yet, right? This is a wonder and an opportunity. Why should we hide or sit in the suck of some weird shame projection? I have more experience now in my life than I've ever had! Why should we be quiet? Let's ask what this time in our lives is *generative of*. What is our body giving to us? How can we use it moving forward? Who might we form community with along the way? How can we bear witness to and record our stories, bring our stories to life, for ourselves and for those who are coming? How do the differences between our stories amplify the diversity of experiences like a giant and beautiful array of voices and bodies? How can we give something to you, readers, and at the same time, inspire you to keep giving and living your truths, to carry on and carry the story and then pass it on to the next person when it is their turn, with bravery and song burst?

Let this blood is mine again become like a body anthem. A love song from us to ourselves, one that reminds us all that we are not at the end of anything. We are at the ever-becoming. Of everything. Flashing our hot without apology.

SECTION ONE
Thresholds

CRONE AGE

By Cheryl Strayed

I was standing in front of the chalkboard of my high school freshman English class delivering an oral book report of Herman Melville's novella, *Bartleby, the Scrivener,* when I first began menstruating. Clad in elephant gray corduroys, I read aloud to my teacher and classmates from the page that quivered in my hands while pretending that a tiny invisible carpenter hadn't set up shop inside my pants, alternately tapping a hammer against the insides of my hip bones or tightening them with a vise. I prayed the fabric of my trousers would be sturdy enough to contain whatever was happening on the other side of it. I prayed I wouldn't blush or blurt out an apology and bolt from the room. But more than anything, I prayed that I was right. That *this was it.* That I was bleeding at last.

I was fourteen, which seemed to me then mortifyingly old to

not yet have my period. In desperation, I'd begun lying about it to my friends, pretending to know exactly what they meant when they complained about menstrual cramps. Occasionally, I even had the gall to complain about them myself—usually to get out of playing dodgeball in PE class. When someone asked me if they could borrow a pad, I'd rummage earnestly around my backpack as if one might possibly be there. Which is a long way of saying that by the time I actually did get my period, on the day of my *Bartleby, the Scrivener* book report, there was no friend to tell. I had to suck it up and handle it like an old pro.

In the bathroom after class, I jammed a wad of toilet paper into my underpants. After I emerged from the stall, I washed my hands and gazed solemnly at myself in the mirror, feeling quietly thrilled by my secret transformation. I was a woman now, at least in one important way.

I wasn't waiting anymore. The next part of my life had begun.

It was decades before it occurred to me that there would be another part after that, or at least another part as far as my ovaries were concerned. Was *menopause* a word I even knew back then? If it was, it lurked only on the far edges of my consciousness, like *pulchritudinous* or *lachrymose*, words whose definitions I'd look up in the dictionary and instantly forget, my use for them close to nil.

Menopause felt so distant to me it was almost as if it didn't exist. Like my life would forever be counted out in rotations of twenty-six days—my cycle being a tad shorter than the norm of twenty-eight, which I knew because I kept meticulous track. On the final pages of each of my journals all through my twenties and thirties and forties, I drew a menstrual chart of numbered grids that I colored in and annotated each month. A record of my life in blood.

It was on these grids that, shortly after my forty-eighth birthday, I noticed something was up. Like the jagged lines on a seismogram that denote the earth shaking far off, my menstrual chart was the first indication of the little earthquakes happening inside of me. Over the next couple of years, my once-predictable cycles wobbled and wavered until they went entirely out of whack. By fifty, they'd become so erratic they couldn't properly be called cycles anymore. They didn't circle around anything. They had no center of gravity. They came and went like the wind or the rain. They were mild or merciless. Torrential or scant. They had a schedule I knew nothing about. It could be twenty-two days between my periods or one hundred and fifty-six.

It was as if I was back to being fourteen again. Wondering when blood would show up in my pants.

It just so happened that during this time—in the months between what would turn out to be my penultimate and final periods—my daughter turned fourteen and, soon after, began menstruating. Ours was a house of hormones in flux, the ground shifting beneath our feet in ways that were both undeniable and undetectable, each of us waxing and waning as we orbited in opposite directions around the same sun. Years before I became a mother I'd imagined if I ever had a daughter, I'd honor her menarche with a ceremonial gathering of all the women who loved her. We'd burn candles and bestow upon her symbolic beads and stones with allegedly special powers and go around the circle sharing words of wisdom and support, welcoming her into womanhood. But by the time I was an actual mother with an actual daughter I knew that if I suggested such a thing, I'd barely get a word out before she said, "Mom, stop."

My own mom—for whom my daughter is named—was menstruating when she died of cancer at forty-five, a fact that outraged me for years, as if it were an insult to her femaleness rather than an affirmation of it. Every organ had shut down except this one—her body decimating itself while her ovaries hummed along as if it were business as usual. It had been she who'd told me about menstruation when I was six or seven, my older sister and I seated on opposite sides of her on the couch as she drew what looked like a bull's head with long draping horns on a notebook in her lap.

"These are your fallopian tubes," she explained cheerfully as she glided her pen across the page. "These are your ovaries. They hold your eggs—every egg you'll ever have is already inside of you. You're born with them. And this," she said, tapping the tip of the bull's nose, "is your vagina."

I drew a similar image for my children—both my son and my daughter—when they were about the same age that my sister and I were when my mom had drawn it for us. And I adopted her tone—the one she used whenever she conveyed information to us about the intimate parts of our bodies or sex—frank and practical and honest, even when it made her blush.

"How old were you when you lost your virginity?" I demanded one day when I was in eighth grade, giggling at my own audacity. My mother couldn't bring herself to say it out loud, but, to my surprise, she flashed the number to me with her hands. Seventeen. And then she answered every question I had about that—the who, where, and why. A guy named Mike who'd been a year ahead of her in school. The back seat of a car on a quiet road in Colorado Springs. Because she thought she loved him.

I was stunned and dazzled and disoriented, the teenage sex life of my mother gobsmacking me into imagining the possibilities that lay ahead for me.

And yet, in spite of these intimacies, I didn't come home that day of the *Bartleby, the Scrivener* book report and tell my mother that I'd gotten my period. I was too embarrassed to share such a private thing with her, my every move during that time designed to distance myself from her, as if I could refuse to let her know me. A few months later, she figured it out on her own. One afternoon when we were driving, she exclaimed with a glimmer of injury, "You didn't tell me you started your period!"

"Why would I?" I snapped back so harshly she went silent.

My own version of *Mom, stop.*

I thought of her a lot in that year when my daughter started bleeding and I ceased to. Having lost her so young—at twenty-two, when I was a senior in college—it wasn't unfamiliar to me to be doing yet another Big Life Thing without her. I'd graduated college two months after she died and a decade later earned my master's degree. I'd written and published my first stories and essays. Married my husband and had two children. Written and published four books. Made a home in three different states she'd never been to. Done a million things that neither of us would have dared to dream were possible. And I'd done them all without her.

But to go through menopause without my mother felt different than the other things. I needed her in that same way I'd needed her as a child and teenager, when she was drawing me pictures of bulls that were actually ovaries and vaginas and telling me about having sex in cars with boys named Mike. I needed her to map it out with me, to tell me her body story, so I could better navigate and understand mine.

When I was studying and marrying and mothering and working and moving to far-off states and making homes, I was always doing some version of what my mother had done before me, even if our versions radically differed. There was no version of my mom in menopause, or even, as far as I know, perimenopause. For the first time, she couldn't be my frame of reference. Hers was not a body against which I could compare my own. I was venturing into territory where she'd never been. I'd grown beyond her, aged years past her. There are so many things my mother didn't get to do or be because she died young, but the one that felt the saddest to me was that she didn't get to be old.

And here I was—*am*—the lucky one. Getting to be.

There's a lot of hard stuff that comes up in perimenopause and certainly plenty came up in mine—hot flashes, insomnia, brain fog, strange facial hair surprises—but all through it, I never forgot my luck. What a gift it was, to simply be there. To laugh and cry and complain about the discomforts. To marvel at the mystery of my very own change of life. Of my body becoming like the wind or the rain, rather than a clock. Of the cycle stopping so I had no choice but to spin in a whirl of my own making. I'd taken to joyfully calling the era that awaited me beyond menopause my Crone Age and in those years of perimenopause as I approached it, I felt the presence of my mother so acutely it was as if I were carrying her along with me past the place where we'd left off. As if I were making good on the promise of every woman whose mother died too young and becoming a crone for both of us.

The word *crone* comes from the Anglo-French word *caroigne*, which means a *carcass or carrion*—literally dead flesh—and modern dictionaries don't improve much upon that, defining the word succinctly as *an ugly old woman*. The Crone Age of my imagining rejects these patriarchal constructs, and draws instead on feminist interpretations that celebrate and affirm the wisdom and power of postmenopausal women. It's not hard to do. The coolest women I know—the ones who'll tell you the truth and love you through everything; the ones who've been there, who know how to be tender and openhearted and also stand their ground—a good number of them stopped bleeding ages ago. To step into the sisterhood of them is *gold*.

By the time I was fifty, my periods were coming so seldom that I abandoned the hand drawn menstrual charts in my journal and downloaded an app called Big Day that counts down the number of days between now and whatever occasion you put in. A birthday. A deadline. A trip. You're officially in menopause one year after your last period and so I added an occasion in the app I titled "Crone Age" and set the date back a year every time another period showed up, until—a month before I turned fifty-three—I reached it. My Big Day.

It didn't occur to me to have a ceremonial gathering for myself, to ask the women who love me to gather in a circle and bestow upon me beads and stones and wise words—and even if I had wanted to do that, I couldn't have because the COVID pandemic was raging. It didn't occur to me to tell my daughter I was now officially in menopause because I imagine she'd have said, "Mom, stop." It didn't occur to me to tell anyone because menopause isn't a story we tell much yet.

Instead, I did what I did all those years ago when I got my first period. I went into the bathroom and gazed solemnly at myself in the mirror, feeling quietly thrilled by my secret transformation. I was a crone now, at least in one important way.

I wasn't waiting anymore. The next part of my life had begun.

UNSILENCING

By Nguyễn Phan Quế Mai

The first time I ever heard a personal story about menopause was in 2003. I was thirty years old, working at the library of the American International School Dhaka in Dhaka, Bangladesh. During our afternoon tea, which took place in a cozy room at the back of the library, Barbara Nicolai—my wonderful German colleague—told our head librarian Beth Phillips and me that she hated the hot flashes, but found it liberating to be free of her monthly period. I was both shocked and amazed: shocked because Barbara would share her personal story so openly, and amazed because I realized I longed for the day I no longer had my period. I had always experienced such bad period pain, so intense that sometimes I felt like fainting. I dreaded my monthly cycle.

That evening, once I was home, I checked for the definition

of "menopause." Reading this, you might think that I was naïve not to have been aware of menopause earlier, not to be more educated about women's health. But growing up in rural areas of Việt Nam in the '70s and '80s, I was surrounded by taboo topics. Discussions about "private affairs" such as menstrual cycles were certainly taboo. Even though I grew up with women around me, my mother, my aunts, and my older female cousins never once mentioned the word "menopause," let alone their menopause experiences, as if it was a shame they had to hide.

THE SHAME

Shame was certainly the feeling that I had whenever it came to my period. Perhaps it was because the Vietnamese word for "period" is *kinh*, which also means "terror," "terrible," or "disgusting." I remember vividly the first time that I had my period: It happened in 1988 when I was fifteen years old. It was a beautiful day and the sun was singing its rays of light down onto swaying canopies of our mango and coconut trees, together with chirpings of birds. I felt the kiss of summer on my hair as I ran free, playing hide-and-seek with my cousins and friends in the garden of my home in Bạc Liêu, a small town in the Mekong Delta, Southern Việt Nam.

"Stop." My eldest cousin, Sơn, suddenly pulled the sleeve of my shirt. His voice was stern. I turned around to meet his serious face.

"Go inside the house." He frowned.

"Why?" I asked, giggles still spilling out of my mouth. I'd

won the previous round of the game by hiding myself inside a gigantic pile of rice straws near the kitchen. Straws that smelled of the golden harvest. Straws that would fuel the hungry flames of my mother's stove as she cooked us one delicious meal after another. For this new round of the hide-and-seek game, my hiding destination was my favorite coconut tree, which stood by the fish pond, laden with fruit. I'd climbed it countless times, enough to know I could swing my body up onto its large, solid fronds and hide myself behind a large bundle of green coconuts. I had to hurry because the seeker—my friend Cẩm—was covering her eyes with her palms, her face turned toward the wall of my home, counting from one to one hundred. She had already reached twenty-one.

"Just go inside!" Sơn snapped at me, his face turning red.

"But why?" I demanded.

"Just go inside and change your pants." He looked disgusted and flicked his hand, the way someone flicked away a mosquito.

Inside the cool bedroom, furnished with a bamboo bed, which I shared with my mother, I took off my pants and gasped: Blood had soaked the seat of my cotton trousers, turning the white and green flowers imprinted on the fabric into a crimson red. Staring at the fresh blood, I felt fear, like a snake, slithering down my spine. No one had taught me about periods. My school lessons had not mentioned it. None of the many books I'd read had covered it. Nor my mother, who worked as a teacher and farmer, and who had told me countless legends and fairy tales. There was no menstruation in such stories.

THE SECRET

The only thing I knew about having a period was that I had to keep it discreet, the way my mother had had to do over the years. We lived in a home crowded with males: my father, my two elder brothers, and my several male cousins who came from my parents' villages—more than one thousand kilometers away—to stay with us to further their education and gain better job opportunities. It was the year 1988 and my mother had no disposable pads, let alone tampons. She had washable pads—rectangular sheets of white cotton fabric that she'd cut from large sheets of fabric she'd bought at our town's bazaar and sewn herself. I knew nothing about her period pain, nor the inconveniences of having a period, only about these white sheets, fluttering quietly to themselves at a hidden corner of our garden, at the very back of our washing line.

So, that day, with my period running down my thigh, I frantically searched for my mother's white cotton sheets. I found them, neatly folded and stacked deep inside her clothing cabinet. I picked one up, fumbled with it, and managed to wedge it between myself and my fresh underwear. It felt chunky. It felt strange. It felt dirty and humiliating, not because I was using my mother's pad, but because I still felt the sharpness of my cousin's words.

THE MEMORY

My mother came home soon after, her body warm and damp with sweat: She'd been laboring on our rice field. She put aside her conical palm-leaf hat and dried my tears with her calloused hands. In a gentle voice, she told me that I should not be afraid nor worry, and that it was natural for a girl of my age to experience menstruation. She explained that I was going to bleed every month, each time for a few days, and she would make new cotton pads for me: I would have my own collection of white sheets. Once I was calm, she collected my soaked pants, underwear, and a white cotton sheet, put them into a brass basin, and showed me how to wash them by hand (we rarely had electricity by then and didn't know about the existence of a washing machine). I was amazed she didn't wince with disgust when she dipped her hands into the bloody water. And then, for the first time, she hung the sheet under the brilliant sun, in the middle of our washing line, as if to declare I should not be ashamed of my body.

Still, my mother, who is now eighty-two years old, did not reveal to me one single thing about menopause. She was likely experiencing perimenopause conditions by then but I'd had no idea about it.

"What was menopause like for you, Mẹ?" I asked her in June 2023, relaxing next to her, both of us sipping the refreshing juice from our green coconuts. We were stretched out on the long chairs that faced the blue, pristine ocean of Phan Thiết, at our favorite beach resort in Southern Việt Nam. By this time I had experienced menopause myself: the hot flashes, the chills, the night sweats, the sleep problems, the mood swings, the joint pain.

"It was so long ago, I don't remember." Sitting on the beach, my mother scooped a spoonful of the soft, white meat from her own coconut and gave it to me. Her answer surprised me. My mother is someone whose memory is better than most: When someone in our family cannot recall a past event, we always turn to my mother.

"Can't you remember, Mẹ? Really?" I asked.

THE STRUGGLE

What I dislike most about menopause is the lack of sleep that it brings. Before I became a novelist, before I was hit by the waves of menopause, I slept easily and soundly, like a rice seed after a harvest, knowing it had done enough work for the day, and it was time to rest, to recuperate, before a new planting season begins. Eleven years ago, when I started writing my debut novel, *The Mountains Sing*, followed by my sophomore novel *Dust Child*, that restful feeling disappeared.

My novels tackle difficult periods of the complicated Vietnamese history and bring to life voices that have been buried, brushed aside, or censored. Those voices would often call out to me during the night, telling me that they could not sleep until I told their stories. Following their callings, I would get out of bed, write furiously for a couple of hours. And as the sun rose, gifting me with its soft light via my open window, I would tear myself away from my writing desk and my computer. I would get back to my bed and curl up next to my husband, who would take care of our children's breakfast and send them off to school. I would sleep soundly for the next few hours, get up and work again. Writing fiction brought interruption to my sleep during the night, but I would almost always catch up with sleep again during the day.

Menopause is different: I wake up during the night, drenched in sweat, unable to fall asleep again. There is no character calling out to me, so even if I drag my body to my writing desk and try to write, I struggle and fail. I return to bed, exhausted. During those nights, I spent many hours in the dark, convincing myself I could go back to sleep, if only I was mentally strong enough. Frustration and disappointment overwhelmed me. I felt disappointed in myself for wasting time, for not knowing how to take care of my health better.

"The hot flashes, the night sweats, the loss of sleep, the mood swings?" Sitting on the beach, my mother repeated my question. She looked out to the ocean, her eyes distant. "Perhaps I experienced them but I can't remember. It was in the early 1990s, and you remember, don't you, how difficult things were at that time? I had so many things to take care of. We had to survive so many things then."

And it hit me that my mother experienced menopause during the most difficult period of our family's history: In the early '90s, Việt Nam embarked on its *đổi mới*—or renovation period, to transform our country from a socialist to market economy. People were allowed to venture into private business, and to trade, hence needed to raise capital. Due to the lack of a well-functioning banking systems, *hụi*, or tontine—self-organized capital-raising schemes where people buy shares of a common fund held by a host—sprang up like mushrooms in a forest after a heavy rain.

My parents, who were teachers and farmers, managed to earn great interest from our savings by buying shares in a tontine organized by a woman whom they trusted. Soon, they began to borrow from friends and relatives to be able to invest more. My parents were assured by the fact that their host had always conducted the business efficiently and was trusted by a large number of people, many of whom were government officials and even members of the police.

I will never forget the day when I was sitting at my desk, studying, next to a window that opened out to look onto our pond. Suddenly I heard someone screaming from our kitchen. The voice sounded like my mother's, but it couldn't be her. She should be at her school, teaching her afternoon class. Dropping my pen and notebook, I ran into the kitchen and saw my mother; she was kneeling, crying uncontrollably. To my shock, she started to hit her head repeatedly against the large clay jar that contained our drinking water.

Once I managed to pull my mother away from the jar, once I managed to calm her, she told me, between sobs, that the host of our tontine had run away, taking with her all of our savings, including the great amount of loans my parents had borrowed. And now, we were left with mountains of debts.

My parents already worked around the clock at their teaching jobs, in the rice field, the garden, and the fish pond, their income barely managed to feed three young, hungry children plus teenage nephews. They had saved every penny for their children's education.

Soon our living room filled with those we owed money. I

remember how loudly they shouted at my parents. "What will you do to be able to earn such large amounts of money?" one woman asked. She knew about my parents' meager salaries and that our rice field was not that fertile.

I grieved for the money that we had lost, knowing how hard I had had to work to help earn it. Together with my parents and brothers, I had labored on our patch of field, digging up bullets. The field used to be abandoned—a stretch of a dike that was used as a practice shooting range for the Southern Vietnamese Army during the American War in Việt Nam. The land was dry as rock and filled with thousands and thousands of bullet casings. My parents, my brothers, and I spent months digging up the metal casings, removing them, ploughing and hoeing the field until the soil began to loosen, ready to receive rice seedlings. On that field, we yielded seasons of rice, sesame seeds, and green peas.

I will never forget those days of hard labor, how my mother's toes splayed out as she walked miles upon miles carrying the water, how the water disappeared into the dry earth, how each grain of rice that we managed to harvest was equal to nine drops of sweat, true to the Vietnamese proverb "*một giọt lúa vàng chín giọt mồ hôi.*" I will never forget how the debtors, after shouting and insulting my parents, decided to take away our belongings. We had no television then, no fridge, barely anything of value except for several pigs and chicken, our three bicycles, and a radio cassette. The debtors fought over them. I wept as they carried my bicycle away.

My mother had to quit her teaching job to try to earn money

to repay our debts. Can you imagine your teacher, one day teaching you in the classroom and the next day, on the street, begging people to buy ice cream? That was my mother. Still, the debts kept piling up, due to the high interest, and the only way out was to sell our house—the house my parents had bought with their life savings.

Upon reflection, I can understand now that the symptoms of my mother's menopause were diluted in the sea of difficulties she was experiencing. She must have stayed sleepless night after night, trying to find the way out for us. And if she sweated profusely, she must have blamed the tropical hot weather, and the fact that we didn't have electricity: When we lived in our house, we rejoiced every time the power was on, perhaps one evening every two weeks, but when we moved after selling the house, no power line could reach us.

My mother had no luxury of consulting a doctor then: She did not have time, nor money. Her health was not a priority: The priority was to keep our family afloat, send the children to school, and repay the remaining debts.

I have always considered my mother a survivor: She survived the French colonization of Việt Nam, the Japanese invasion, the Great Famine during which approximately two million Vietnamese died, the American War in Việt Nam, which tore our country apart, and the war's aftermath. Perhaps it is because of her survival instinct that she's chosen to forget about menopause.

Could it be that unprivileged women are more likely to silence their menopause experiences, thinking that these are not valid or should not be prioritized? I imagine myself to be one of the millions of women currently living in emergency situations created by wars and armed conflicts around the world. I imagine myself to be one of the many women who risk their lives crossing deserts or oceans to reach freedom, to pursue a better life for their children or for themselves. If I were one of these women, I would be unlikely to mention menopause when you ask me about the issues I face.

I have interviewed Vietnamese women who spent their youth in jungles during the war. They all told me about the ways they tried to evade American bombs, to search for food, to survive Agent Orange that was being sprayed onto them—a chemical that has proven to be poisonous, causing cancer and birth defects. None of them shared with me how they'd managed their menstrual cycles. One woman, however, did share that due to stress and poor nutrition, her period did not appear for many months.

My experiences have taught me the importance of unsilencing the menopause experiences from those who have had to bury them. Every woman, regardless of their social position, has a story that is valid, unique, and worth listening to. And stories about menopause should be a part of personal and collective history. Stories about menopause are mirrors that reflect a society's political, social, cultural, economical, and medical aspects. Only when we normalize the discussions about menopause among underprivileged groups can we enable help to reach them more effectively.

THE INJUSTICE

I once blamed stress for the absence of my period. I was forty-seven years old at that time, living in Indonesia and about to relocate to Kyrgyzstan. Living the life of an expat seems exciting and it is, but it also comes with a great deal of heartache. The act of uprooting myself and my family was so stressful and painful that I did not notice my period had stopped during the first two months. Later on, I convinced myself that it had stopped because of my stress. I refused to acknowledge that my menopause was arriving. I expected my period to reappear. When it didn't, I began to worry, especially when the hot flashes, the chills, the night sweats, the sleep problems, and the joint pain were intensifying.

Kyrgyzstan is not known for good medical facilities, and I don't have a gynecologist, also because of the language barriers (people speak either Kyrgyz or Russian). So it took me a whole year to talk to a doctor about my menopause: I was back home in Việt Nam and went to a private clinic for an overall health checkup. There, I told a female doctor about the conditions I was experiencing. I asked her whether I was having menopause and what it meant for my body. I was especially concerned because my fingers had gotten so swollen that both my engagement ring and wedding ring became too small, they hurt me badly, I couldn't sleep at night. I had spent days trying to take the rings off, first using cream, then soap, then fine strings; when none of them worked, I had to go to a jewelry store where a technician cut them apart.

My doctor looked at me. I couldn't read her facial expressions because they were hidden behind her COVID face mask.

"Menopause," she said. "It means you are aging, your productive system has withered!" Earlier, when I was having an ultrasound with a gynecologist who worked in that same clinic, she showed the image of my ultrasound to an intern, saying: "See the patient's ovary? It has shriveled."

In recalling the exact words the doctors had used that day and writing them down now, I am furious at how insensitive they were. When I left the hospital, I was shocked and dazzled. My menopause had been confirmed. It hit me, for the first time. For years, I had been thinking that one day, maybe one day, I would have a third child, the way my mother had had me after my two brothers.

And now, it was too late.

I detested the way my body had been described by my doctors, as if I was defined by my birth-giving capacity. And for the first time, I realized that I needed to learn as much as possible about menopause, about its many myths and misconceptions so that I can use this knowledge to take care of my health and help my Vietnamese female friends.

THE RESEARCH

The more research about menopause I did, the more I realized the need to unsilence the menopause experiences of all women, regardless of our circumstances, so that we can create equal access to health care and counseling.

I found out that in Vietnamese, the term "menopause," *mãn kinh*, means the period runs out. The Wikipedia page and websites of several reputable Vietnamese hospitals define *mãn kinh* as *"giai đoạn quá độ từ tuổi trung niên sang tuổi già* (menopause is a period when the body proceeds from middle age to old age)." Menopause almost always has negative connotations. It is often only linked with aging. The scientific articles that I encountered rarely associated menopause with freedom, the way my librarian friend, Barbara Nicolai, had described it to me twenty years ago.

It is true that menopause can have adverse health impacts on women. Research done in Việt Nam on Vietnamese women confirmed that "middle-aged women often encounter a wide range of both physical and psychological health problems when approaching menopause, most commonly vasomotor symptoms, mood changes, sleep disorders, and sexual dysfunction…Menopausal symptoms can become distressing."[*]

During and after menopause, women's ovaries produce very little estrogen. According to the US Department of Health and Human Services, this change can raise the risks of heart disease, stroke, osteoporosis, lead poisoning, urinary incontinence, and cavities.[†]

My current doctor, the one I trust, has kindly told me that the symptoms of menopause can be managed by an active, healthy lifestyle. In my prescription, she wrote: "Forty-five minutes of exercise every day." She gave me suggestions regarding what vitamins I should take.

---

[*] Thao Thi Phuong Nguyen et al., "Determinants of Health-Seeking Behaviors Among Middle-Aged Women in Vietnam's Rural-Urban Transition Setting," *Frontiers in Public Health* 10 (2023), https://www.frontiersin.org/articles/10.3389/fpubh.2022.967913/full.

[†] Office on Women's Health, "Menopause," https://www.womenshealth.gov/menopause.

The knowledge I gained from my research about menopause has led to significant changes to my behavior. Every day, I make an effort to consume foods that boost estrogen: fruits such as apples, berries, grapes, grains, nuts and seeds, tofu, and vegetables. I regularly go out in the sun to get vitamin D. I exercise daily, as I know that exercise is one of the best weapons to combat the symptoms of menopause.

For me, I know that menopause is a period of time that demands I pause and reconsider how I can take better care of my health. And that I can enjoy the freedom that it gives me: no more period pain. No more pads or tampons. I can exercise every day without my period bothering me, and at any time, I can plan for a holiday to the beach without having to look up my menstruation calendar.

I turned fifty years old in August 2023, and I have not had my period for a few years now. I feel good. I still wake up during the night, yet I have found that a good dose of exercise and taking a magnesium supplement the previous day, as well as deep breathing, will help me go back to sleep.

Now I cannot live without my daily sport. These days, thirty minutes of intense exercise can be easily done from the comfort of one's own home, following an online routine, or a yoga session readily available on YouTube. If the weather permits, I love running on the street. I walk everywhere. And I swim.

Menopause has taught me to become my own healer. I know now that sleep is important, therefore I aim to go to bed early. My family, my better diet, my exercise, my vitamin intake, my laughing yoga, my friends, and my books are my daily medicine.

THE RENEWAL AND TRANSFORMATION

I have arrived at a place where I refuse to accept that menopause is a body's decline. I was never a runner but I started running in 2023 during my book tour, when I was fifty years old. At the beginning of 2024, I came first in my age group in a five-kilometer run, as part of the Hồ Chí Minh City Midnight Marathon. I am still riding the waves of my menopause; and the experiences have not always been pleasant, but I am grateful for the lessons.

I am being transformed into the next phase of my life.

Menopause is a period of renewal and transformation—a new beginning. I am a new person now: and I am more than my ability to give birth. I am more than my physical body: I am my strong will, my determination to make each day on this earth meaningful.

THE UNSILENCING

Unsilencing has been one of the missions of my writing: to unsilence trauma that has been buried, brushed aside, or censored. Through unsilencing our difficult experiences, we can validate them and acknowledge that we are worthy of being listened to, hence find solidarity, community, and healing.

Yet unsilencing difficult experiences is not an easy process. It often faces rejections, as I did countless times when I tried to publish my debut novel and first book in English, *The Mountains Sing*. This novel includes rarely documented experiences of Vietnamese people in world literature, told via the viewpoints of Vietnamese women. Many agents and publishers who rejected my manuscript thought that the story was "too sad," "not uplifting enough." Yet I didn't give up looking for a publisher for my book because I felt speaking about suffering— of any woman—is the portal to changing the collective history and allowing healing to take place.

It has been challenging to write this essay since I had to relive the many painful experiences of my past. In detailing the mistakes my parents once made about their investments, I worried I was betraying them. In the Vietnamese society, filial piety duty— the duty to show loyalty, love, and respect to one's parents—is of utmost importance. However, during the process of reflecting and writing this essay, I could sit down to talk to my parents about those difficult years, and realize how hard they had worked to pull us out of the bottomless abyss of debts, and how they had refused to give up hope. I was reminded of how many ice creams and baskets of vegetables my mother had sold, how many buckets of water my father had poured onto our rice field and garden, how many mountains of earth he'd dug, so that my brothers and I could go to universities. In writing this essay, I understood my parents' unconditional love for me, and how they never failed to believe in me. We are still deeply traumatized by what happened, yet our conversations have facilitated healing.

Once I finished this essay, I could look back and understand a little bit more about myself and the people around me. I found solidarity with my parents and with the very first reader of this essay: my literary agent—Julie Stevenson. Julie was the only agent who believed that the sad stories in my novel, *The*

Mountains Sing, needed to be told. After reading my essay, she reminded me that it is an important perspective to include the experiences of encountering menopause during times of war and social upheaval. She wrote: "I, too, had little information about perimenopause and menopause here in the US, and the information I got from doctors, even female gynecologists, was not sufficient or helpful…For me, it was important to learn to trust my own intuition about what I felt my body needed because the Western medical establishment has some catching up to do when it comes to truly understanding women's bodies."

Julie's comment surprised me. Living in a developing country sometimes makes me think that the medical system in the West caters better for menopause issues, even though I deeply respect and regularly practice the Eastern medicine philosophy. I hope that we can find a way forward where we can combine the Eastern wisdom and Western medical science when it comes to dealing with perimenopause and menopause.

On that day at our favorite beach resort, when I spoke with my mother about menopause, she scooped the soft, white meat from her own coconut and gave it to me. My mother has never said she loves me, she simply expresses it by giving me her food: nourishment.

By writing this story and by being part of *The Big M* anthology, I am hoping we can find more ways of nourishing one another. By unsilencing our experiences, reaching out to embrace one another's stories, we can feel less alone, more seen, more informed, more assured, and more empowered.

THE MENOPAUSAL GARDENER'S ALMANAC

By Reyna Grande

I'm a woman of a delightful season.

—*Sandra Cisneros*

ISSUE #1: NOT EVERYTHING IS PEACHY

I have a peach tree in my garden. In November, as the days shorten and the air turns crisp, she sheds her leaves and readies herself for the winter, a period of dormancy when she must conserve her energy and prepare for what's to come. Then it's spring, and like me, from the moment she awakens, she gets to work.

Delicate pink petals burst forth from her buds, marking the end of winter. The blooms, fleeting and beautiful, leave a carpet of pink on the ground and make way for the new leaves of spring. And then, the baby peaches appear, tiny and full of promise. I watch them with a mixture of anticipation and protectiveness.

I'm a self-taught gardener. Much like my writing, what I know about gardening is mostly from trial and error. And I've erred plenty. With my peach tree, my error is greed.

As the baby peaches grow, I'm delighted at the tree's abundance, the potential of all that fruit. I know peaches need to be thinned when they're the size of a thumbnail, but discarding some of the fruit feels wasteful. So, I betray the tree and leave all the fuzzy green babies cradled on her limbs. I dream of cobbler, sauces, and jam. I get my grill ready and buy a dehydrator.

By June, as the peaches become plump, branches begin to bend or break under the weight. The fruit is smaller than it should be, overcrowded, and competing for space and nutrients. Heavy with fruit, the tree sags, its branches bearing the weight of its abundance, looking utterly, beautifully, tired.

I recognize that look.

———

When I was twenty-six, I had a baby with a man fourteen years my senior. I wasted $3,000 taking him to court to get him to pay child support. In the end, I carried the burden of financially supporting myself and my son and bore the sole responsibility for his well-being.

An emergency teaching credential allowed me to work at a middle school. The teacher shortage created this opportunity for me, for which I was grateful. A bachelor's degree in creative writing hadn't prepared me for a "real job," and now I had a baby to provide for. I taught during the day and took classes at night to earn a more permanent teaching credential. In between teaching, studying, and nurturing my child, I was also writing a novel.

I woke up at dawn and went to sleep past midnight. Every hour became a task to be a "productive" mother, woman, writer. Did I have the strength? To stay grounded, to bear fruit, to bend, not break, as I strained for the sun? Every ounce of effort was demanded.

One sweltering afternoon, the air thick and heavy, a storm erupts with high winds. Pelting hail, the size of marbles, clashes against the roof, a rare and unsettling occurrence for our usually gentle summer. I worry about my peaches, which aren't yet ripe enough to eat. When the sky clears up, and I go outside, there are dozens of peaches on the ground. I lament the loss of the fruit, but as I gather them in a bucket to throw them into the compost bin, I realize that Mother Nature has done what I could not. She removed the excess weight off the tree, and by doing so, took a load off me as well. It was then that I felt the full force of my greediness at wanting to take too much from my tree. To have overburdened a mother, to have exploited her fertility and fruitfulness and forced her to carry more than she should.

At thirty-two, I got married and became a mother for the second time. My daughter took her first flight with me at two months old. The year before, I had committed to doing an event at a conference in the Bay Area. I couldn't pass up the opportunity. It would put me in contact with thousands of educators who worked with English learners, immigrant children, and children of immigrants. It was the perfect place for me to speak about my recently published novel and get it into the hands of these teachers. I knew too well that my book wouldn't succeed by the grace of God, my publisher, and the media.

So, I decided to fly up there with my baby cradled in my arms. I was breastfeeding her and couldn't leave her behind. And what would my husband do with a two-month-old? He would already have his hands full with my six-year-old son. At the same time, I didn't know what I would do with my baby during my presentation.

The only people I knew at the conference were my fellow panelists—so I couldn't ask them to babysit during our event. As I walked around the exhibit hall, searching the crowds for someone I recognized, my daughter started crying. Her wails resonated in the exhibit hall. A teacher conference was no place for a baby. But what else could I do? A voice in my head replied: *You should have stayed home with your baby instead of trying to promote your writing. What a bad mom you are.*

Luckily, Jose Luis Orozco came to the rescue. He had a booth showcasing his children's song books and CDs, a well-loved resource for teachers. Kids loved him. I had never met him before, but he was a friendly man. He picked up his guitar and started singing "Juanito cuando baila." The exhibit hall became his stage. As he serenaded my baby, she fell back asleep, lulled by his beautiful music. Briefly, I considered asking Jose Luis Orozco if he would watch my daughter, but as I saw him surrounded by his customers, I decided he had his hands full already with his booth. Plus, hadn't I just met him? Still, I was getting desperate.

As we were being led to the presentation room, I encountered a familiar face: Mrs. Wrinkler, a teacher from Santa Cruz High School. Ten years before, during my undergraduate studies at UCSC, I had taught creative writing to her English Language Learner class. Recognizing her instantly, I implored her to babysit my daughter during my presentation.

"I have an appointment, but I can spare twenty minutes," she replied, accepting my sleeping child.

The presentation began, with my fellow authors taking their turns. Time, as it often does in such situations, sped by. Before my turn arrived, Mrs. Wrinkler signaled from the doorway, her time up. I quickly excused myself from the stage, thanked her for her brief assistance, and returned to the podium with my baby.

I did most of my presentation with Eva bundled up like a burrito in my arms. I clutched her close, her tiny body a warm weight against my chest. Her breath, soft and steady against my neck, the scent of baby powder and milk mingled with the nervous sweat on my palms. I felt so unprofessional. *What must those teachers be thinking? Were they judging my choice to drag my baby with me here when she should have been home, sleeping soundly in her own crib? Would they not take me seriously?* Cradling my daughter, I talked about my book, my immigration journey that had inspired the story, and my experiences as an English learner in California public schools. While I spoke, I kept praying my baby wouldn't wake up.

Perhaps lulled by my voice, she slept through the entire event, even the Q & A, and when the presentation was over, I was physically and emotionally exhausted.

As we were leaving the room, a woman approached me and introduced herself. "I'm from the city of Watsonville. I'm on the committee that chooses the book for our city-wide read, and we are considering your novel. It's so nice to meet you!"

I returned home from the conference with a heavy weight: the sense that I had prioritized my writing over my children. But weeks later, I received the news that Watsonville's book committee had chosen *Across a Hundred Mountains* for its program. In addition to purchasing books, they were paying me to visit the area. This lifted some of the guilt I'd been carrying.

Finding a balance between nurturing my writing, taking care of my children, and maintaining a happy home was—and is—a constant challenge. There are days when the weight of dirty dishes and unanswered emails threatens to topple me, when the blank page on my computer screen reminds me of my failure to nurture a story to fruition. The guilt, the self-doubt, the constant questioning—*Am I doing enough? Am I giving enough? And I producing enough?*—can be overwhelming. But occasionally, good things happen that alleviate some of the burden and make the load I carry easier to bear.

After a particularly wet winter, the following spring my peach tree is infected with a fungus called *Taphrina deformans*, which causes the leaves to grow large and swollen, then curl and distort. I pluck the infected leaves off the tree, but they are too numerous, and soon they wither away and fall off on their own, leaving the branches mostly bare. The baby peaches that emerge barely cling to life. My tree is sickly and distressed, yet she still works hard to produce and be fruitful. Carry on.

———

My forties are marked by a series of health issues that worsen as I age. Not long after I celebrate my fortieth birthday, I'm diagnosed with keratoconus, a condition that is making my corneas lose their shape. It causes blurriness that glasses cannot fix. Later, my eyesight gets even blurrier, and I begin to suffer from dry eye—a common symptom of menopause.

Then, I am also diagnosed with hearing loss. I noticed it was becoming harder to understand questions and comments during my presentations. I often have to ask the audience members to repeat themselves. When watching TV with my husband and kids, I keep asking, "What did they say?" Putting on the subtitles doesn't help as much because of my weakened eyesight.

At forty-four, while getting off the train, I tear a ligament on my right knee and have to use crutches, then do physical therapy. My knee has weakened, and at times it feels as if the joint is held together by a brass paper fastener, like those arts and crafts projects from elementary school. At forty-six, I develop sciatica, which makes it hard to sit for long periods of time. My brain begins to associate writing with physical pain. When I travel for my speaking engagements, I endure hours of discomfort while strapped to my airplane seat, unable to move. Sometimes, I can't sleep because of the sciatic nerve pain radiating from my glutes to my feet.

When my productivity diminishes, I blame my middle-aged body for betraying me.

These physical changes are accompanied by emotional and psychological shifts too, a sense of loss and a need for adjustment, like my peach tree adapting to a new season.

When I'm hit with bouts of depression over my health, the writing doesn't come at all. Meeting the needs of my children and my husband, and working hard to provide for our home, feels overwhelming. But for too many years, I've learned to measure my days by my productivity, by how much I can accomplish by the end of the day. Now the less I do, the more I feel like a failure. Who am I if I can't produce? If I can't create? If I cannot bear fruit?

~

Trees cannot heal their wounds in the way we do. They cannot regenerate or repair cells. Instead, they grow new wood over the wound to enclose it, to isolate the injury from the rest of the tree. The wound isn't healed, it is sealed and contained. This keeps the pathogens in the infected area from causing further damage, protecting the tree. I think about this when I prune my peach tree. Every cut leaves the tree vulnerable to infection and decay. But pruning is essential to the maintenance of a tree. If done correctly, it extends its life, helps it conserve resources, gives it better shape and form, and best of all, strengthens its core. All this will lead to tastier fruit.

As my tree grows around her wounds, surviving her injuries, I think about my own wounds, and how I have learned to compartmentalize my trauma, sealing those wounds but never quite healing. Like most, I will never get over my trauma, but I learn to live with it and learn to adapt, to grow around the pain.

—

It's spring again, and my peach tree is sprouting new leaves and beginning a new fruiting cycle. This time, I will better protect this mother tree and spare her from exhausting herself. When the time comes, I will go out to the garden and thin her branches, not regretfully, but with gratitude for the abundance she offers. I will lighten her load, allowing her to focus on nurturing the remaining fruit. And when those peaches come into their ripeness, kissed by the sun and nourished by the earth, they will be sweeter for the care and restraint that allowed them to flourish.

I realize that this new stage in my life, my middle years, might be an opportunity for regrowth. This is a time to release the need to prove myself endlessly, to stop being greedy with my body's resources, and instead, to offer it the care and kindness it has so long deserved. I will learn to thin my own metaphorical branches, not with regret, but with a new understanding, focusing on what truly nourishes me. My body, marked and changed, is a testament to a life lived fully, bravely, and with heart. As it enters this new season, in exchange for fertility it is offering me a hard-earned wisdom, a clearer vision, and a gentler strength.

ISSUE #2: THE QUEEN'S LAMENT

"How will I know if I'm starting menopause?" I ask my doctor at my annual physical.

One of the telltale signs of menopause is a woman's menstrual period. It becomes irregular until ovulation ceases. The problem is I haven't had a period in over fifteen years. When my daughter was born, I got an IUD, which stopped my menstrual cycles altogether. At forty-six, after continuing to replace my IUD every five years, I think it is a good question to ask my doctor. If I don't get my period, how the hell am I supposed to know if I am truly menopausal? And would suppressing my menstrual cycles for all these years come back to bite me in the uterus?

My doctor is a tall white man in his mid-sixties. I feel intimidated by his presence, but I push myself to express my concerns about the changes in my body. I tell him about the nights I've woken up drenched in sweat. At first, I tried to put a positive spin on the night sweats. *Hey, my body is burning calories and detoxing while I sleep! What's so bad about that?* The reality was, waking up soaked and restless is disturbing. It's something happening to me without my control. I also have been feeling hotter than usual, although that might not signal hot flashes. I've always been warm. My daughter has always loved to cuddle with me because she says I'm "warmer than a thousand suns."

I tell him about the ache in my hips, my wobbly knee, my

struggles with my eyesight, my hearing, acid reflux, carpal tunnel, sciatica, and so forth, but as I hear myself share these things, I worry about sounding like a hypochondriac. I'm too embarrassed to tell him other things that I find too personal to share, like, when I cough or sneeze, I leak a little.

"Let's do some blood work," my doctor says.

As the lab technician pricks me with his needle, and I watch my blood gushing into the sample tubes, I wish I'd done a better job advocating for myself, asking more questions of my doctor about menopause and the best way to handle it. *Based on my symptoms, how do I know what stage of menopause I'm in? What kind of changes should I look out for? Any warning signs I should be aware of? Are my night sweats and feeling hotter than usual consistent with hot flashes related to menopause? Could the aches and pains I'm experiencing (hips, knee, etc.) be related to hormonal changes during menopause? What about my worsening eyesight and hearing? How might the symptoms be connected?*

When I return from a speaking event out of town, I make my rounds of the garden and notice something unusual. Above the side porch by the orange tree, I see bees going in and out of a small crevice in the wood. I tell my husband we should keep an eye on it. "Those bees are up to something," I tell him.

A few days later, I look out the glass dining room door and see a swarm of bees flying on the other side. Thousands of them. I can hear them buzzing. I can almost feel the vibrations. The only thing standing between me and those bees is a pane of glass. For a moment, I wish I could open the door and stand out there, let them settle on me, welcome them to my garden. Except, they cannot stay. They chose the worst spot to make a home, right outside the side door. I search for a beekeeper who can come get them.

—

I receive a message from my doctor about my blood work. It reads, "The hormone levels do confirm menopause."

I guess it's official then.

The email says nothing else. No explanation about what the blood work results indicate about my hormone levels and how they relate to my symptoms. Nothing about what I'm supposed to do now. How to take care of myself or what lifestyle changes I should make to better manage my symptoms. Nothing on what to expect as my body changes. No resources or recommended follow-up appointments. I want him to reassure me. I feel that I am about to begin a journey into an unknown country where I have to learn a whole new vocabulary.

—

I find a local beekeeper who does humane bee removal. He comes to assess how big the hive is, where the queen bee might be, and how to get her out. He thinks she might have left her hive to start a new one. This piques my interest.

"Why do you think she did that?" I ask. What factors caused her displacement?

"She probably got too old. The new queen would have killed her if she'd stayed."

I think about my doctor's appointment, as I sat in the sterile lab and watched my blood being drawn, a torrent of questions swirling in my mind: "What stage of menopause am I in? What kind of changes should I look for?"—these same questions come back to me when I face the bees. Am I, too, a queen that's gotten old?

———

My name means queen in English. So, I feel a certain connection to anything "queeny." In this case, I become obsessed with the secret lives of queen bees—their vulnerable power, their challenges of aging, and the threat of replacement. The bees become a metaphor for my own fear.

In the articles I read, I learn how perilous the queen bee's position is and how it gets worse with old age, just like human females. When the queen bee's fertility wanes and her egg-laying ability is compromised, the colony will breed a new queen who might then sting the old one to death, unless she makes her escape, taking her followers with her.

Sometimes, it is the hive itself that kills its queen once it decides to reject her and replace her to ensure the survival of the colony. The bees will surround her en masse. "Balling the queen" is the term beekeepers use. This ball of bees will raise the queen's body temperature until she overheats and succumbs.

In other words, they give her the ultimate hot flash.

～

The beekeeper shows up with a vacuum to suck up the bees. "You'll kill them!" I say, suddenly protective of my new hive.

"I won't harm them," he promises. The vacuum is specially designed to store the bees in a bucket, alive and well. I watch with fascination as he climbs up a ladder and begins to smoke them out.

Soon, the vacuum is turned on, and as I watch the bees get sucked up and put into the bucket, a wave of unexpected sadness washes over me.

"Are you sure it's safe?" I ask him again, and he shows me the bucket so that I can see the bees are not being injured or killed.

It isn't just about losing the bees, but the uncertainty I feel about my own changing role. Like that queen bee displaced by a new generation, am I also being subtly "removed" or replaced in some way? This isn't just about nature or my garden, but about the nature of being a woman navigating midlife, a time when our bodies shift, and societal expectations often make us feel we're no longer needed in the same way.

When the beekeeper is done, he takes my bees and their queen away to give them a new home and gives me their small honeycomb as a keepsake.

～

In her poem, "At Fifty I Am Startled to Find I Am in My Splendor," Sandra Cisneros celebrates the beginning of this decade in a way that I hope I will feel when I am fifty, which won't be long now. She writes, "I am Venetian, decaying splendidly / Am magnificent without measure."

I also love the haunting beauty of ruins. And like Cisneros, I would like to feel magnificent in my fifties. To embrace the changes that come with time. To age with intelligence, grace, and dignity. I yearn for a life free of the patriarchy's sting. When the time comes, I hope to have the courage to take flight and escape before it kills me.

———

Being sick or physically injured is a death sentence for the queen bee. Mites can attach themselves to the queen and feed on her blood. A fungal or bacterial infection can lead to deformities in her brood, or even death. If one of her legs is injured, she cannot as easily roam around the honeycomb, limping along as she tries to lay eggs in the cells. Surviving in a world where they live a perilous existence, an underperforming queen who cannot fulfill her duties could be a death sentence to the colony.

Supersedure, the replacing, then takes place.

———

Reading about the queen bee's "supersedure" hits a nerve. That sense of being replaced, of being seen as no longer essential— it echoes the very anxieties I have about entering menopause. In the same way the bees decide when their queen's time is up, does society, in some ways, dictate when a woman's prime is over? It makes me question who gets to decide our worth, and when.

I fear I am not doing a good job of "decaying splendidly." My forties have kicked my ass health-wise, and I worry about what my fifties will bring. All these health problems have caused panic, and I don't have the resolve to push against society's unrealistic standards of beauty and perfection. I feel like I'm coming undone. I worry I am at risk of not being useful. Am I underperforming? Will I let my family down?

I give in to the pressure of keeping aging at bay. Even if it's just superficial, I find ways to slow it down. I use henna to dye the gray in my hair. I buy expensive face creams and sunblock. I even give Botox a try. As I sit in the dermatologist's office and wince when the needles sting my forehead again and again, I think of the bees killing their old queen.

And for a moment, I feel that there's a part of me that's dying.

———

Queen bees rarely sting humans, reserving their venom for other queen bees. Usually, when queens meet, they will fight to the death. Even when the colony breeds new queens to replace the aging one, the first to emerge will often kill its unhatched rivals. In the human world, this behavior has been twisted into the "Queen Bee syndrome," a harmful myth that women in power actively suppress other women. This idea, perpetuated by the patriarchy to divide and conquer women and make us turn against each other, is a dangerous mindset that promotes a scarcity mentality.

Yet my journey from undocumented immigrant to college graduate to professional writer has been defined by women who have uplifted me, guided me, and helped me take flight. These women actively reject the patriarchal narrative. They've shown me a different path—one where new queens and old queens not only coexist but thrive together. They've shown me that I have it in me to redefine what "splendor" means at this stage of life. My body holds stories, and those stories are invaluable.

———

Turning forty-eight, I seek a fresh start with a new doctor. It's time to move on from the towering white male figure who always made me feel like I couldn't fully express my worries. My choice this time is a woman of color, someone older who can likely empathize with my journey through menopause. This decision fills me with hope that my future concerns won't be met with a dismissive attitude, but with understanding and guidance. Most of all, I will no longer feel that I'm being a drama queen.

Instead of fearing "supersedure," I choose to embrace this new chapter as a powerful evolution. I'm not a bee to be cast out, but a woman stepping into her strength and wisdom. My aging is not a lament, but a celebration of the life I have lived and the queen I am becoming in my own right.

ISSUE #3: IT'S MY SLUG PARTY AND I'LL CRY IF I WANT TO

"I'm depressed the way a slug-ridden cabbage might be expected to be," wrote Samuel Beckett. His words echo in my mind as I take in the devastation in my garden, a slug-ridden testament to my despair.

The slimy trails, the gaping holes in my kale and Swiss chard, the decimated strawberries. Seedlings that sprout one day and are gone the next. It's enough to make any gardener weep. Desperate to protect my babies, I research how to get rid of the slimy creatures without using pesticides. The suggested methods are cruel, but when our plants are threatened, gardeners can be brutally protective—hunting them down and cutting them in half with scissors; drowning them in soapy water; spraying them with ammonia; sprinkling them with salt; putting them in a container and shoving them in the freezer. Since slugs and snails are cannibals, another suggestion is to crush them and leave their corpses as a trap to attract more of them to the slaughter. Some gardeners prefer to eradicate them with beer. A boozy demise, a final fiesta before the eternal sleep.

I buy a case of Mexican beer at Costco. If Mexican beer can conquer the US market, then maybe it can drown a few slugs.

With beer bottles in hand, I set up my slug bar and place bowls throughout the raised beds and the flower beds and fruit trees, fill them to the brim with beer and wait for the fiesta to begin.

———

Slugs and snails are hermaphrodites, which means they have the fascinating ability to self-fertilize, but that would reduce the gene pool, so they usually avoid this. According to the *Old Farmer's Almanac*, the average garden contains more than fifteen thousand slugs and snails. Being hermaphrodites, each slug and snail can lay eggs, so if they are *all* capable of becoming moms, how much beer will I need to buy? Or better yet, how long will it be before *this* mom starts drinking it herself out of frustration?

~

Between 10 p.m. and midnight, instead of cuddling with my husband in bed, I roam my garden, armed with a flashlight and a stick. My bowls of beer are surrounded by slugs and snails, who are having a blast in the cool night air. The trick with the beer is that they'll get drunk and fall into the bowl to drown. But for some, the beer isn't as effective. Instead of waiting for them to get wasted enough to fall in on their own, I use a stick to help them to their happy death. Then I return to bed, where my husband is sound asleep. I lie awake for hours, just me and night sweats. And I feel like going back out to the garden with the slugs and snails and letting the damp, midnight breeze cool off my sticky body.

~

The snail has an exterior shell, which means it carries its home on its back. But they are not born with it. Little by little they build it with calcium found in the soil. Only when its home is finished is a snail old enough to engage in romance.

~

When I met my husband at twenty-eight, though I was technically the more "experienced," I was far from feeling fully realized or liberated in my own body.

Most of my previous partners had been one-night stands or fleeting affairs; one was even without my consent. Men who toyed with my feelings, bedded me, and moved on. What could I possibly learn from that? I rarely had orgasms. I was too nervous or felt too guilty to enjoy it. The truth is most of those encounters were the result of my childhood trauma. Having grown up with an alcoholic, physically abusive father who was emotionally unavailable, my need for closeness and approval forced me to find love and attention elsewhere. Did I learn to enjoy sex from those encounters with men who were replacements for my father? I think the opposite happened. I felt dirty and used every time I traded sex for a bit of affection.

I carried the shame and regret of my past sexual encounters into my relationship with my husband, preventing me from experiencing deep intimacy. I was unable to be truly comfortable with my body, being honest about my needs, my likes and dislikes. I wanted to be a good lover, for our lovemaking to be satisfying to us both, yet I'd developed a complicated relationship with my sexuality and felt unclean, vulnerable, and afraid of not being worthy of him.

———

Beneath the moonlight, I'm captivated by the mating rituals of slugs and snails in the garden—a slow, deliberate dance of connection that unfolds in the cool night air. When they are in heat, the slime of slugs and snails contains pheromones that let the others know they are on the prowl. All the horny slugs have to do is follow the slime, and a slippery seduction ensues. When two lovers find each other, the foreplay can last for hours. They nibble and wiggle, they bite, they entwine. Theirs is a mating ritual of mutual pleasure and reciprocity, where they exchange sperm with a partner. After a nocturnal tryst, feeling equally satisfied, the two lovers go their separate ways to both become mothers.

———

In our younger years, there were times when my husband reached for me, and I was too exhausted and preoccupied to respond. Teaching, wrangling the children and taking them to their extracurricular activities and doctor's appointments, cooking, cleaning, gardening, and then squeezing in precious time for writing plus the occasional book reading and school presentation was utterly exhausting. Those nights when my husband needed me, I didn't exaggerate when I said I was tired. Bearing the burden of housework and childcare leaves most women with little energy for intimacy. I suffered anxiety over this, internalizing it as a personal sexual failing. The fear of disappointing my husband, of making him feel rejected, haunted me.

This sense of inadequacy has followed me into my middle-aged years, where my complicated relationship with desire and sexual angst is now compounded by the changes brought on by aging and menopause.

———

The Greek god of fertility, Priapus, was a protector of plants, gardens, and penises. According to the myth, when he was a baby, he was cursed by Hera with giant genitals. Perhaps slugs and snails have also incurred Hera's wrath. Their penises are as long as their bodies. Proportionally, they have the largest penis-to-body ratio in the animal kingdom.

Sometimes after mating, if they have trouble disengaging from their slippery embrace, a slug will chew their partner's penis off, or their very own. This is called apophallation. The amputated slug lives out the rest of their days as a female. Making them more vulnerable to predators and infections.

—

The mascot of my alma mater, UC Santa Cruz, is the banana slug. The campus is nestled in a redwood forest, the habitat of *Ariolimax californicus*. Students take pride in being slugs and embrace the uniqueness of our mascot. The summer before my senior year, I got drunk while hanging out with two other of my fellow slugs. I was a lightweight and passed out after a few beers. I woke up in the middle of the night and found one of my friends on top of me, inside of me. I closed my eyes and willed myself to fall back asleep. Pretended it wasn't happening to me. Afterward, I never called it rape. I called it my stupidity. I didn't blame him. I blamed myself. *By drinking with him, hadn't I invited the assault?*

Now, I wish I had turned him into an apophallated slug. I wish I had liberated myself from the patriarchy's culture of victim-blaming that made me believe it was my fault.

—

Slime is the secret weapon of slugs and snails. It helps to deter predators and protects their fleshy skin from desiccation, keeping it moist and supple. Above all, the slime of slugs and snails is the surface on which they crawl across the ground, protecting their soft, vulnerable bodies from sharp things, making them capable of crawling unharmed across razor-edged wire.

—

Lately, I've been noticing that when my husband and I make love, my vagina has become increasingly dry, leading to painful sex. This is yet another way a woman's body changes because of menopause. We produce less estrogen, which in turn leads to a reduction in vaginal secretion, which means the vagina does not get properly lubricated.

In other words, menopause is making my vagina feel like a slug desiccating in the sun.

Though some of us women experience a decrease in our sex drive in our middle-age years, a surprising fact I learn in my research is that the less sexually active a menopausal woman is, the more likely her vagina will change, becoming shorter, thinner, and less elastic. To prevent vaginal atrophy and dryness, it is recommended that we continue to have sex on a regular basis to keep our vaginas thick, flexible, and moist.

So it's either use it or lose it.

It occurs to me that my nightly slug hunting might be detrimental to my vaginal health.

—

Slugs and snails aren't the only ones enjoying their slime. A component in their secretions is mucin, which contains allantoin, glycolic acid, hyaluronic acid, and peptides, ingredients used by the skin-care industry. Mucin is the new beauty trend, with companies making "miracle" products that contain snail slime—face masks, cleansers, creams, and serums. Mucin is said to improve hydration, increase collagen production, and rejuvenate skin cells. In their reviews, snail-mucin devotees gush over their new skin glow.

When looking in the mirror and seeing the fine lines, wrinkles, and age spots on my face, I wonder if it's time to put the beer bowls away. Instead of crawling all over my garden, should I invite my slugs and snails to crawl over my aging face?

~

As we say goodbye to our forties, I've noticed that my husband and I are both experiencing the physical changes that come with age. Reaching for each other sometimes feels different now. We're both figuring out how to navigate the shifts in our bodies and energy levels. I feel less alone knowing that I'm not the only one on this journey of hormonal changes, decreased libido, and persistent fatigue. As we navigate menopause and andropause as a couple, my husband and I are learning to adapt together to these new physical changes and shifting desires. Menopause, surprisingly, has forced me to confront those long-buried inhibitions and sexual traumas. It's pushed me to be more honest with my husband about my needs, to seek new ways to connect and redefine intimacy both in and out of the bedroom.

My vagina, once a place of shame and too long ignored, is now demanding attention and care. I've never had to work so hard to keep it happy! Of course, a good bottle of lube will also help.

Perhaps the silver lining to these challenging times is the growing empathy my husband and I have for each other as we strive to be kinder and more supportive.

So, as I give up on my garden night patrol and put the beer bowls away, I reflect on the lesson learned from watching my slugs' tenaciousness, their strange mating rituals, and their ability to leave a trail of protection. After twenty years together, as my husband and I navigate this new landscape of our lives, may we, like those garden slugs, find ways to adapt, to protect each other, and to create our own shimmering path forward together.

FROM MENTAL PAUSE TO POWER SURGES

By Joey Soloway

What is mental pause? Ohhhhh, this essay is supposed to be about men-o-pause. When I was a kid I used to think it was "mental pause." I thought that when you got older you would just pause. Thinking. Because your brain would be too crusty and crunchy. And then you would go into your mental pause.

At some point, I realized that mental pause had nothing to do with menopause and got old enough to menstruate with vigor. Now I think back about when I did have my period, and I—oh periods. What a fucking hassle. Just thinking about them makes me seize up.

My therapist Ellen Silverstein (who has since passed away but who holds the title "The Great Ellen Silverstein") used to say the whole reason that there was such a thing as misogyny and patriarchy is that men saw women bleeding with the moon, and realized that we have more power than they do.

Meaning the power to tell time—a literal wall calendar—resides within all of our actual assigned female at birth bodies. These awful men must have shoved one another angrily, wondering: Exactly HOW could it be that some people and the moon could be in such perfect rhythm? But yet we were. Women were.

In addition, we bled without dying, which must have been real cool and utterly intimidating. And thus, men started a campaign to make us hate ourselves.

—

It's not until you finish having your period that you realize how disgusting and horrifying your period actually was.

I think I've blocked out the four straight decades of repeated incapacitation. And now that I no longer menstruate, when young women come over I find them to just be absolutely revolting. I walk into the bathroom and suddenly there's piles and piles of tissue in my garbage, meant to cover something bloody at the bottom. My dog finds their spongy, spongy materials and immediately chomps into them like so much Gaines-Burgers, then leaves them all over the house.

Why can't we feel better about our menses? Men have so many different kinds of super heroes, but all we got was Wonder Woman, Bionic Woman, Superlady, and I think I'm making some of these up. Why isn't there a Period Lady who can attach a neat fitting onto her labia so that it can extend into something like an elephant's trunk and spray her enemies with her very own high-powered Red Tide?

        ⁓

I worked hard to hold on to my self-esteem even though as I entered adolescence it was clear that getting your period was a major effing hassle. Such a hassle it would be better to just sit everything out when you have it. How is it possible that every three-and-a-half to four weeks, so much blood and other kinds of fetal material (including things that were spongy and livery)—would come out of our vaginas in a rush? Not just for a few minutes or a few days, but sometimes multiple days of gooey, chunky, jello-y ooze. Coming out of me like a gash! Like a war wound!

Sometimes during the days that the rivers of blood were rushing out of me onto those fat white diaper pads lodged in my underwear, I would start to feel angry. Anything could make me seethe and then boil over. Like the sight of men playing pick-up basketball.

I mean FUCK, not only did women not get to do anything with other women remotely like this public ritual of careening our sweaty bodies into one another, but in addition, we also had a gash between our legs that spat thick blood out at least one out of every four weeks.

Yes, I was bleeding all the time, I was bleeding 25 percent of the time, one in four days I went through pants and underpants, pads and pads and more pads, makeshift pads out of those brown paper towels in your high school bathroom.

Even worse, I was so horny. Horny like clockwork. My best

friend and I used to give each other a knowing wink and say, "Day 17?" Day 17 was the seventeenth day of your cycle, when you were sure to get pregnant, and you were so horny you would fuck the corner of a table. Or a bookshelf. Or anything nearby, even if it didn't mean to impregnate you. You just wanted it in ya. That's Day 17. Day 15 and 16 you're more flirty than imaginable and you want to go out and meet people, even if they're gross. Hoping that they're going to impregnate your egg, which is surely coming. Then on the seventeenth you're willing to have sex with anybody, even if they're a bookshelf, a bookcase, a table, a table saw, a band saw, or that gross guy from that bar in that band.

We didn't have Plan B then, we just had Days 18, 19, and 20 of regret and shame. Wondering how it was possible that we could have seen so much potential in that gross guy's eyes. Day 21 and 22 and 23, all was lost. I'd want to be in my menstrual hut or some sort of a cave where I didn't have to see people. And if anyone came near me I blamed them for things they couldn't possibly have done.

I'm old now, and with the wondrous mix of Lexapro, testosterone, and Who Cares Anyway, I don't cry much. But boy did I cry a lot on the days before, during, and after my period. In fact, if I was out in the world on Days 21 or 22 you could be certain I'd get into an argument with a cashier and be weeping before my things were bagged. "Stay indoors on Days 20 to 21 to 22!," I would tell myself!

And then it would all start all over again, believe it or not. Monthly! In tune with the moon. We ARE magic!

I recently found out that the later you get your period, the earlier you go through your mental pause, aka menopause. You would think it would be the later you get it the longer it goes for, but in fact, people either have a short menarche or a long menarche. And I, apparently, had an uncommonly short menarche. I only menstruated from the late age of sixteen and stopped at around the early age of forty-four. Now that's a short menarche! Thus, if you do your math, you will find that I have been in full mental pause for a good fifteen years, from forty-three to fifty-eight.

I got pregnant with my second kid at the age of forty-one, nursed my kid for a year, and my period never came back. A couple of years later, I started to have hot flashes. They weren't combined with any other symptoms, just plain old hot flashes. I was finally annoyed by menopause. I went to my therapist, the aforementioned Ellen Silverstein, and complained.

My hot flashes felt like they were powered by shame. Sometimes I'd be in a pitch meeting and I would realize that I was having a hot flash. Sweat beads would start to form on my upper lip and the next thing I knew I'd be asking for a wet paper towel midway through the meeting. Being a mom and trying to be appropriate in meetings was already hard enough. I remember once I pulled a used diaper out of my computer bag and set it out on the table instead of my iPad. Hot flashes felt like that kind of shame.

I complained to Ellen about my hot flashes. I said to her, "In the middle of the night I can get out of bed and jump into a cold shower and get back in bed, but when it happens in the middle of a meeting—I just don't want to be that person. It's so embarrassing."

"Embarrassing!" Ellen Silverstein said. "You know what I call hot flashes?"

"Tell me, Ellen," I said.

"I. Call. Them. Power surges."

"Power surges?" I thought. Now this was interesting!

She said, "We have so much power throughout our lives. Women have so much unnoticed, unnamed, unseen POWER. And as your body starts to not have to work so hard to get what you want, you get older, you get more confident, you get more aware of what your boundaries are. What you deserve. You know how to say what you want. These hot flashes are actually little surges of power—your electrical system going BOOM! POW! FLASH! FLICKER! FLOCKER! FUCK ALL Y'ALL I AM SO ABOUT TO BE OUTTA HERE BAM!"

I started to imagine, in this room full of people, that my power was my own, whether or not I carried a doody diaper around with me, whether or not I had the ample bosom and the moist skin of a young woman, whether or not I had my mental faculties or in fact needed to take many mental pauses. This sweaty fountain, this little light of mine, I'm gonna let it flow. These power surges. Watch me go.

SECTION TWO

Mapping the Body, Mapping the World

A BRIEF BUT DETAILED HISTORY OF MY UTERUS

By Nana-Ama Danquah

I am traveling on rough road when I see the sign.

"Rough road" is what the locals in Ghana call a street that's unpaved. Usually, it's a pothole-riddled strip of red dirt. Sometimes, if you're lucky, it'll have been covered with a thin layer of black gravel, pieces of rock so small they get caught in the tread of your tires. It's 2012, well over a year since I moved back to the country of my birth. I am a local again, accustomed to navigating this terrain.

The sign reads: OLD LAYERS FOR SALE.

By the time the words register, I am already down the road, past the large shed-like structure on whose door it is hanging. I can't tell you how many times I've seen that sign, how many times I've driven past, carrying the weight of those words with me throughout the day and on into the night. It makes me sick, the thought of those chickens who'd spent their entire lives laying eggs only to now be cast aside.

I make a split-second decision, then a sudden U-turn, leaving a plume of dust in my wake. I park crookedly in front of the place, my front tire inches away from the open gutter. My stride is brisk and once inside the shop, I stand there, my heart beating so loudly I can feel the vibration in my ears.

For months, I've been wanting to come inside but now that I am here, I feel silly. The sense of urgency fades into uncertainty. Why am I here? What do I intend to do? I don't know, I don't know. I take a deep breath. The air smells, predictably and pungently, like chickens. It's an indoor coop. I can see the birds, packed several to a cage. The cages are tall; they are made of wood and mesh wire and stacked two stories high. My eyes lock onto a single white feather falling, slowly, majestically, to the ground.

The back door opens and a man, silver-haired and slightly bent, shuffles slowly down the narrow aisle between the two rows of cages. He approaches me, says "Good afternoon," then follows with, "How many do you want?" He sounds exhausted; not from the day, which is still young, but from life. Trickles of sweat are forming rivers inside the dark creases of his skin. I wipe the back of my neck, in solidarity. Accra is a humid place. The shed has no air-conditioning.

I hear myself, voice shaking, asking the man why they are selling the layers. I purposely omit the word "old." He looks at me as though the answer is ridiculously obvious. Still, he responds courteously, tells me they're of no use to him now because they're no longer able to lay eggs. I know this already, yet hearing it out loud brings me to tears. The man seems startled.

"Do you know what a layer is?" he asks, avoiding eye contact. Before I can say anything, he is talking about feed and water and eggs, which are supposedly those birds' sole purpose.

"They're just old hens now," he concludes. "Even their skin is too tough for any food other than soup, and you have to let it keep on the fire for long."

I feel myself unraveling, on the verge of exposing a part of myself I have kept hidden beneath perfunctory smiles and social politeness, a second self who is fed up and rageful. I turn on my heels and rush through the door. By the time I am in the car, that second self has fully emerged. She is bawling, punching the steering wheel, not caring when her fist smashes against the horn and it blasts a loud, menacing sound. The man rushes outside to investigate. There is a look of horror on his face as he stares at the wild woman sitting in her vehicle, swinging her arms, fighting a seemingly invisible enemy. That wild woman has been kept at bay for the last few years. That wild woman is me, and I am her. We blend now, become indivisible.

I think about the chickens, the old layers, and the fate that awaits them. I think about every time I've heard someone refer to a woman as a chick or a hen, or used a chicken's dissected anatomy to describe part of a woman's physique. I think about the various ways in which we women are also caged, our bodies turned into objects meant only to meet the requirements and needs of others. I think about how, when we cross the threshold of a certain age and our bodies are no longer of use to others, we step straight into invisibility. We, too, become disposable.

This thought returns me to my body, myself. There are fibroid tumors in my uterus. If I graze my fingers along the skin of my lower abdomen, just above my pelvic area, I can feel them. It's 2012. I am forty-five. In four years, I will undergo a partial, or supracervical, hysterectomy. Already, I bleed for half the month. On those days, my bedroom resembles a crime scene. I wake up in a small pool of blood; there are smears and spatter on my thighs and on the sheets, in the empty space next to me where in some alternate universe, a partner sleeps, their chest rising and falling with each soft snore.

I know what's ahead for me, for my uterus, and the fear of that shift is almost too much to bear.

In her book, *Women Who Run with the Wolves*, Clarissa Pinkola Estés writes: "There is a time in our lives, usually in mid-life, when a woman has to make a decision—possibly the most important psychic decision of her future life—and that is, whether to be bitter or not. Women often come to this in their late thirties or early forties. They are at the point where they are full up to their ears with everything and they've 'had it.'"

That day inside the chicken coop in Accra is, for me, the beginning of that time.

———

In December 2001, during my mid-thirties, I had two surgeries. The first was a laparoscopy, which my gynecologist, Dr. Woods, performed in order to see how many fibroid tumors I had, and determine how large they were. The procedure was also used to officially diagnose the endometriosis, which, for years, had been wreaking havoc on my body. It's a disease that causes the endometrium, the lining of the uterus, to grow outside of the uterus, resulting in a host of issues, from adhesions to infertility. Every month when I bled, it caused an excruciating, mind-numbing pain, one that would find me doubled over in bed, a hot water bottle to my abdomen, counting the hours until I could pop another extra-strength pain pill.

Dr. Woods informed me that my uterus was a "mine field" of fibroids, ranging in size from grapefruits to peas. Fibroids are tumors, made up of muscle and connective tissue, that grow inside the uterus. They're usually, though not always, noncancerous. They can cause back pain; frequent urination; a distended abdomen; pain during intercourse; heavy, lengthy periods; and infertility. He recommended a hysterectomy. I flatly refused. He was young, just a few years my senior, Chinese American, with a thick head of hair that was black as tar and so shiny it looked synthetic, as though it belonged on the head of a doll. He and I spoke casually, honestly. Our relationship was absent of any doctor-patient formalities. We had history.

"You've had your child," he said, the implication being that I was no longer in need of a uterus. That made me immediately defensive. My fists clenched, yet I kept my tone jovial, almost joking.

"Oh, I'm still young," I reminded him. Indeed, I was only thirty-four. "Who knows what the future holds."

"You're planning to have another baby?" Dr Woods asked, his eyes widening. His shock and concern were palpable—and they were an appropriate response. Exactly one decade earlier, while he was still a resident, Dr. Woods had helped me deliver my only child. During the sixth month of my pregnancy, I'd been diagnosed with preeclampsia, a life-threatening complication. Among the symptoms of preeclampsia are uncontrolled hypertension, protein in the urine, and other signs of possible kidney damage. One might also experience elevated liver enzymes or other signs of liver damage, fluid in the lungs, blurred vision, nausea and vomiting, shortness of breath as a result of fluid in the lungs, debilitating headaches, sudden weight gain, and water retention resulting in extreme swelling of the hands and feet.

In the beginning my symptoms were not severe; mostly, I felt fine. The condition progressed. By the time I was told that my baby would be delivered early, my blood pressure had skyrocketed; the headaches were, quite literally, blinding; I could not walk a short distance without getting winded; and I'd gained a tremendous amount of weight. My face and extremities were so swollen I was nearly unrecognizable. A few days before my due date, labor had to be chemically induced.

For a long time, I assumed that the reason I didn't fully appreciate the seriousness of that condition was because I was young. Even though Dr. Woods had told me that labor had to be induced because if I didn't deliver the baby right then, I would die; even though several times during my thirty-six-hour labor I'd begged him to shoot me between the eyes and put me out of my misery; it was only after my daughter had arrived and they'd lifted my body, placed it onto another gurney and wheeled me into the intensive care unit that I fully understood how dangerously close to death I was, and had been, teetering. The truth is that no one, not even Dr. Woods, had properly explained the gravity of my circumstances. I had not been given medication. I was simply told to rest and limit my stress.

In the United States, the maternal mortality rate of Black women is disproportionately high. For every one hundred thousand live births there are seventy deaths. That is nearly three times higher than for white women, who experience twenty-seven deaths per one hundred thousand live births and for Hispanic women, who experience twenty-eight deaths for the same number of live births. As of this writing, the hospital where my daughter was delivered is the subject of a federal civil rights investigation for its treatment of Black women who give birth in their facility, a disproportionate number of whom have died. When I read this, I was reminded again of how lucky I was to have lived through that experience of childbirth, and how lucky I was to have left the hospital with a healthy baby.

This I know for certain: Dr. Woods single-handedly saved my life. He shut down his colleagues who insisted that I be given a cesarean section. He challenged his superiors who wanted to perform an episiotomy. They all came into my room, wanting to cut me open in one way or another, and he would not let them. He stayed with me throughout the entire ordeal. He was a good doctor, a skilled doctor, a compassionate doctor, but he was also a male doctor. He was a man who now, ten years later, wanted to remove my uterus.

"Even if I never have another baby," I began, "I still want to know that I can. I want that possibility. I want to keep my uterus." I then looked at him, defiance in one eye, surrender in the other, and whispered, "Please."

"Okay," Dr. Woods agreed, scribbling something in my file. "We'll do a myomectomy instead."

What kind of society have we created where a woman has to provide an explanation and then beg a doctor for permission to keep her perfectly functional reproductive organ? Sadly, it's the same kind of society in which an insurance company—a group of people, the majority of whom are usually white, usually men— can refuse to cover any procedure other than a hysterectomy.

At that time in my life, I was not financially stable; I didn't have private insurance. My health needs were covered by Medi-Cal, California's public insurance, a program similar to federal Medicaid. I was suspicious of their insistence that I have a hysterectomy. The procedure wasn't a medical necessity in my case so why were they making it mandatory?

"I'm sure it's because I'm Black," I complained to Dr. Woods. He cocked his head, rested his cheek against an outstretched index finger while cupping his chin with the other digits. He looked at me as if to say, "Go on...I'm listening."

When a Black person suspects something is happening or being done to them because of their race, non-Black people often need to be convinced beyond any reasonable doubt. The problem is that racism is not reasonable. Though racism itself defies logic, one of the reasons it persists is because of people's reliance on logic to prove its existence.

"This is a forced sterilization," I said, scooching my chair closer to his desk. Something I'd long admired about Dr. Woods was that he never spoke to patients while they were on the examination table, legs in stirrups, or sitting ass-out in a johnny gown. If there was a discussion to be had, it'd be in his office with both parties clothed.

He sat up and folded his arms across his chest. "Forced sterilization? But why would they do that?" he wanted to know. "What could they possibly gain from it?" I didn't answer. What could I say to make him believe as unequivocally as I did that Medi-Cal's decision had everything to do with the fact that I was Black, female, and poor?

What I know now is that Black women are three times more likely than white women to develop fibroids. Black women are also three times more likely than white women to receive hysterectomies, many of which are medically unnecessary, as the result of a diagnosis of fibroids. Black women are four times more likely than white women to suffer complications post-surgery that require hospitalization. Black women also have morbidity associated with both hysterectomy and myomectomy that is 50 percent greater than white women. They die from issues resulting from blood transfusion, wound infection, and sepsis.

Whether or not Dr. Woods believed that race was a motivating factor in Medi-Cal's decision remains unclear. He was, however, confident that they had overstepped. They did not have the authority to dictate to him, the physician, the correct course of action for his patient.

"I am going to appeal the decision," he said calmly. "It's not their place to tell me what's best for you. I'm your physician." Thrilled though I was to hear him say that, a part of me was also resentful that he and the officials at Medi-Cal could even hold the power to decide what was best for my uterus. So much so that their wishes trumped mine.

Whatever Dr. Woods told them worked. Within two weeks, I was in a hospital, on his operating table, having the second surgery—a myomectomy, for the removal of only my fibroid tumors.

~

The color of the legal pad I am writing on is canary yellow. It says so on the package. This makes me think of the bird, which makes me think of singing and music, which then makes me think of all the songs I've sung or listened to while some guy was on top of me, his hips thrusting, his breath heavy and warm against my neck, smelling of cigarettes or weed, cheap beer or sweet fruity wine coolers. There've been many men. I am promiscuous, and I don't know why. I will learn many years later, in therapy, that promiscuity is one of the myriad compulsive behaviors linked to childhood sexual abuse, that it is actually a classic coping mechanism employed by many survivors experiencing PTSD.

When I find myself flat on my back like that, I listen to whatever song is playing in the background—Anita Baker, Lionel Richie, Bruce Springsteen, Cyndi Lauper, John Cougar

Mellencamp. If nothing is on, I sing one in my head until the guy is done, zips up, and leaves.

I am writing a list of everyone that I have ever had sex with. Given that I am just sixteen, it's relatively long, though not into the double digits. There are a lot of encounters with the same guys. My mother is forcing me to write this list because I am pregnant. I am a whore, she tells me over and over, a filthy whore. I finish writing the list and leave it on the dining table for her to find. The list is accurate. Almost. There is one name missing—Jonathan. He sexually abuses me regularly and has since I was in the seventh grade. It doesn't occur to me that my mother knows this is happening, that the sole reason she is demanding this list is to look for his name on it. When I am in my twenties, I will discover that she believes I initiated the sexual activity, that I seduced her boyfriend, even though I was a preteen and he was a thirtysomething-year-old man.

I am not yet privy to any of this information, but even without it, I know that she hates me, blames me for everything wrong in her life. She is razor-tongued and mean; she treats me with disdain, tells me often enough that she wishes she'd never had me, that without kids she could have been somebody. It is 1983 in the Washington Metro Area, the place to which my family immigrated from Ghana, barely ten years back. At this age I am still drawn to my mother as home. I am still yearning for her love, plotting ways to be better, to do better so that I am worthy of it.

My period, which will eventually turn textbook, is currently erratic. It comes early, it comes late, it comes exactly on time. I don't keep track, but obviously, my mother does. She figures out that I could be pregnant before I even realize I am late, much later than I should be. She enlists the assistance of her cousin, Gertrude, who stops by the house one evening. Gertrude is a plump, ebony-skinned woman who wears too much drug-store makeup. Her eyes and cheeks and lips are always adorned in garish shades. Gertrude is a medical doctor. She is a quack. I am aware, from several overheard conversations, that being treated by her is a risky proposition. In five years, Dr. Gertrude, as she likes to be called, will be stripped of her medical license and convicted for Medicaid fraud. She will eventually leave the United States and travel to one country after another to set up shop. In each one, she will lose her license for either malpractice or fraud.

When my mother summons me to the dining room and tells me that Dr. Gertrude is going to draw my blood, I nearly faint. I am afraid of needles and I am afraid of Dr. Gertrude, who takes what looks like a large freezer bag from her overstuffed purse. Inside the freezer bag are the tools she will be using. I see an assortment of butterfly needles, alcohol wipes, tubes, and what look to be large rubber bands but I soon find out are tourniquets. Rather than a proper sterile environment, this blood draw will be taking place at a table where a chicken and rice dinner has just been eaten.

For the next ten minutes my arm becomes Dr. Gertrude's personal pin cushion. She slips the butterfly needle into the crook of my left elbow. Nothing happens. She turns it to the left and then to the right hoping to hit a vein. She removes the needle, slips it into another area in the crook of my arm, and repeats what she did the first time. Again, there is nothing. She does this same thing about four or five times. Nothing, nothing, nothing, nothing at all. Finally, she unknots the plastic tourniquet and lets it fall from my arm. She takes my hand, looks at the veins on the top of it. She turns my hand over, then looks at the veins on my wrist, below my palm. Dissatisfied, she moves over to my right arm, thumps two fingers against the inside of my elbow several times, then ties the tourniquet around my bicep, and reaches for the needle. I start crying. It feels like I am being tortured and there is nothing I can do about it, there is no one to help me. I am sobbing so hard I can barely breathe. My mother tells me to shut up and let Dr. Gertrude finish what she is doing. My wails soften into whimpers. On this arm, it only takes a few punctures for the bright red liquid to flow into the collection tube. I watch as it fills. Dr. Gertrude removes it, attaches another tube, and fills that one up, too.

The test results don't arrive for days. When they do, I am not the first to know. I am never actually informed. There is no discussion, at least not with me. I hear my mother making phone calls. Each conversation is brief. I hear my name during each one, so I know it's about me, and the possibility that I'm pregnant.

We are not one of those television families on the shows I tune into every night. We are an African family, insular and old-school. We don't sit around the living room and share our feelings. Parents don't seek permission or approval from their children. Childhood, for me, is a sort of serfdom, complete with berating and corporeal punishment as a means of domination. My mother tells me that I will get an abortion the following day. This is how I learn that the test was positive, I am definitely pregnant.

At the clinic, ten or so anti-abortion protesters with signs line the sidewalk by the front door. When my mother and I pass them to enter the building, a few yell "baby killer," "murderer." One screams, "Don't do it. Don't do it." My mother warns that if she sees any tears or if I behave as though I am in physical discomfort after the procedure, she will beat me. I sit in the reception area, with its standard-issue navy blue armchairs and fluorescent lights, while she goes to check me in. Atop the side table next to my seat is a mountain of various pamphlets. One catches my eye. The cover is split into two blocks; the top is hunter green and the bottom is white, with a splotch of red that resembles a large blood stain. In white print, atop the green and red colors, are the words *No woman is required to build the world by destroying herself.* Underneath the quote, in black print, is the attribution: Rabbi Sofer, Nineteenth Century. When I glance up and see my mother walking towards me, I quickly grab the pamphlet, fold it in half once and fold it in half another time, then slide it into the front pocket of my jeans.

The surgical procedure I am having is a D & C, dilation and curettage, which is used to scrape the uterus clean of any tissue that's inside. It's minimally invasive, done with local anesthesia. This doesn't mean that it's not without its risks. The person performing the D & C is my mother's friend, Dr. Kamau. I know this because I've been to the clinic with her before. During those visits, I stayed in the car while she picked something up or dropped something off.

Dr. Kamau is tall, bespectacled, and slender, an East African who, true to stereotype, has the build of a long-distance runner. He is also a quack, though at the time, I'm unaware of this. Within the next six years, he will perforate the uteruses of several women, perform an incomplete abortion on a woman, and cause the deaths of two other women; one will bleed out on his table and the other will suffer severe brain damage yet hang on to life for three more years before succumbing to her injuries. Dr. Kamau will surrender his medical license in order to avoid any substantive punishment.

While on the examination table, my feet in stirrups, I observe Dr. Kamau picking up what looks like a needle.

"Are you going to give me an injection? Inside my vagina?" I am horrified.

"It's an anesthetic for the cervix," he explains, matter-of-factly. "It's a small needle. Don't act as if you haven't had bigger things in there." There is a moment or two of disbelief, during which I replay his words. How can a doctor speak to a patient in such a vulgar and disrespectful way, I wonder, before remembering that in his eyes I am not a real patient. I am the filthy whore daughter of the woman who spends Sundays drinking with him and his wife. Who knows what he has been told about me to make him behave as though I am not deserving of respect, care, and tenderness. Shame spreads through me like lava as I lie motionless, singing "Sweet Dreams" in my head along with

Annie Lennox, my legs wide open for my mother's friend to extract the contents of my uterus.

~

In the four years between the day at the chicken coop in Accra and the day of my hysterectomy, I attempted to shrink the fibroids naturally. Weeks after my visit to the chicken coop, I returned to Los Angeles to confer with Dr. Woods. Surgery wasn't an option, not yet, not until I'd ruled out every other method of healing. There were teas and other concoctions that promised to melt the tumors away. There were dietary changes that included an increase in my consumption of fiber and cruciferous vegetables, as well as a decrease in sugar and red meat. There were essential oils, herbs, supplements, lots and lots of supplements. I tried grounding, castor oil packs, and Maya Abdominal Massage. I tried to exercise regularly and vigorously. I tried and I tried but nothing worked. It wasn't that the treatments were ineffective, nothing worked because I was never fully compliant. My professional schedule was unpredictable and hectic, making it virtually impossible to remain consistent with any regimen.

For years, I'd been working as a ghostwriter in order to afford my life. There were bills—rent, tuition, clothing, extracurricular, food, insurance, utilities, medical and car expenses—so, so many bills to pay. I ghostwrote everything from letters, newsletters, speeches, book proposals, and full-length books for politicians, business executives, interior designers, health and exercise coaches, self-help and spiritual gurus. I would have ghostwritten their grocery lists if they'd paid me to. The money was good, but it was soul-crushing work.

I found it difficult to reconcile myself with the idea that my writing was worth more when sold with another person's name on it as the author. My writing received all the attention, accolades, and critical acclaim I'd ever dreamt it would, except I no longer owned it. None of that praise or success could help me build my own readership or further my literary career in any way other than as a ghostwriter for yet another project with no recognition. Every book I wrote for someone else was one that I did not write as myself with my name on the cover as the author.

Time, the waste and disregard of it, was always an issue when I was working as a ghostwriter. My time was deemed less important than the client's. Time zone differences found me taking meetings and calls at all hours. I was often stood up, made to wait for inordinate amounts of time, and had meetings canceled at the very last minute. In order to meet deadlines, I habitually pulled all-nighters. And I traveled so much the airlines started inviting me to concerts and sports matches that they sponsored. After my hysterectomy I received "get well" flowers from a couple airlines, and several flight attendants I'd befriended came to visit me.

After a year of false starts and flubs, I realized I could not take a natural healing journey on my own, so I cleared my calendar, drove south to San Diego, and checked into a private health retreat that offered a three-week body-mind-spirit program. I'd heard that it involved eating a raw food diet, having daily enemas, and drinking lots of juiced wheatgrass and rejuvelac, a fermented drink made from sprouted grains. No part of that sounded appealing to me. But I'd also heard stories of attendees who'd reversed illnesses, from diabetes to terminal cancer. I desperately needed that kind of miracle. I was a hot mess—smoking a pack of cigarettes a day, taking pills in order to sleep, eating restaurant and drive-through food, and being crushed under the weight of chronic anxiety. My abdomen was so distended I looked five months pregnant, and I was now bleeding heavily for three weeks of each month.

Week one at the retreat, I went through nicotine and caffeine withdrawal: headaches, irritability, and intense cravings. I felt terrible, but I lost ten pounds!

Week two, I was brand-new, with a pep in my step on morning walks. The bleeding had stopped. It was the closest thing I'd had in years to a regular period. When I'd checked into the retreat to deal with the fibroids, the "body" component of the program had been my sole interest. Much to my surprise, the "mind" and "spirit" classes drew me in. I came to understand that the body must heal as a whole. I was willing to do whatever it took, so I signed up for spiritual counseling, as well as an energy session, whatever that was.

I was assigned a dynamic woman, Amy, to facilitate my spiritual counseling. Long before she'd started working at the facility, Amy had been a guest. She'd been diagnosed with stage IV uterine cancer, which had metastasized in a number of her organs, most notably as a large tumor in each of her lungs. It was the recurrence of a cancer she thought she'd beaten with chemotherapy, radiation, and the removal of her uterus. She recalled to me the first time her oncologist had told her she was cancer-free. He'd said to return to her life, to resume whatever it was she'd been doing before the cancer had interrupted. "But if nothing changes," Amy told me, "then nothing changes."

The cancer returned, and this time, there was nothing more medical science could do for her. Amy heard of the health retreat from a stranger. She checked in and stayed, as many attendees do, well beyond the official three-week program. Several weeks into Amy's stay, after an appointment with her oncologist, she learned that the tumors in both of her lungs had shrunk significantly. At the end of sixteen weeks at the retreat, Amy's oncologist once again declared her cancer-free.

In our first meeting, Amy spoke about how we store emotions and traumas in our bodies, especially our organs. She explained that from a spiritual perspective, illnesses of the uterus usually correlate with silencing, the absence of voice, and/or the suppression of creativity.

"What do you do for work?" she asked.

"I'm a speechwriter and a ghostwriter. I've been doing it for about a decade or more now."

"Are you credited for the things you write?" I shook my head.

"Do you write and publish your own work?" she wanted to know. I shook my head.

"Not really." I rubbed my forehead, let out a heavy sigh. "I just don't have the time. There are only so many hours in a day." She looked at me and smiled. She seemed a bit taken aback by my responses. Even so, her demeanor was gentle, her tone nonjudgmental.

"It looks like you have some decisions to make," she said. "As you're making them, just bear in mind that if nothing changes, then nothing changes."

The next evening, I went for my energy session. In the room, I disrobed, climbed onto a massage table and covered myself with a plain white sheet. The practitioner was a middle-aged Latinx woman who looked like Sophia Loren. She first gave me a massage. After that, she moved on to the energy work, which involved rubbing her hands together as though to create friction and then holding them, palms down, about six inches over my body. She began at my feet then worked her way up ever so slowly. I looked at her, standing there with her eyes closed, intently channeling...what?...energy? *Riiiiight!* Having lived in Southern California for most of my adult life and successfully dodged numerous attempts at recruitment into cults, I like to think I have a well-developed bullshit meter. And that, I decided, is what the energy session was: bullshit.

Energy work, or Energy Healing as it is formally referred to, is based on the concept that energy flows through every living thing in the world, that there is a field of energy surrounding each of us. It's a concept that exists in numerous cultures. In China that energy is called "chi," in India it's "prana," in Japan it's "ki," in several indigenous West African cultures it's the divine power within you. Illness is thought to stem from an imbalance or blockage in your energy field or flow. Energy Healing is meant to clear those blockages so as to advance the body's processes of healing.

I found it fascinating to watch the practitioner work. Sometimes she held her hands stiffly, sometimes she made these graceful, undulating movements, like small waves. Other times she'd glide them from side to side in a subtle sweeping motion that engaged her hips and entire upper body. It was relaxing to watch her swaying to the soft strains of music coming from the speaker. In this way, she inched up from my ankles to my shins, to my knees, to my thighs.

As her hands moved over my thighs, the temperature in the room became uncomfortably warm. When her hands were positioned over my pubic area and pelvis, a scalding heat traveled through my body. It felt like someone had injected a hot liquid into my veins and it was making its way through my entire system. I closed my eyes and for a moment, I was back on Dr. Kamau's examination table. When I opened my eyes, the energy practitioner was right there, her dark brown hair brushing her shoulders each time she moved her hands. My tears fell sideways, landing in my ears. Not a sound came out of my mouth.

When her hands drifted over my lower abdomen, a bolt of electricity shot through me, from my toes straight up to the top of my head. I have never been struck by lightning, but I imagine it would be a more intense version of what had just happened. I sat up straight and screamed, "Stop!" My body was shaking. I was scared. "Why?" I asked the practitioner through my sobs. "What have you done to me? Why?" She lifted her hands, which had been at her side. I thought she was going to continue the session. "No, no, no, no, no, no," I cried, bringing my knees to my chest and leaning away from her. "Please stop. Please stop." She reached her hands out and pulled my upper body into an embrace, letting me rest my head on her bosom and weep until I was all cried out.

"My dear," the practitioner said, "you've got work to do. But you can heal; know that. Have faith in that."

Week three, I was nearly twenty pounds lighter, a non-smoker, with skin that glowed. Best of all, when I touched my abdomen, I could no longer feel the fibroids.

Listen: My life is not a Hollywood movie with a main character who learns some powerful lessons, has an instant transformation, and proceeds to make all the right decisions to fix her broken life.

I did not go home in search of an energy healer near me. I definitely did not continue giving myself enemas, eating raw food, juicing, and drinking wheatgrass and rejuvelac. And most regrettably, I did not fire all my clients, then write a bestselling novel.

A couple of the changes from my time at the retreat stuck. I took regular walks and I never returned to the habit of smoking, but all the other habits I'd kicked came limping back. Before long, I was pulling all-nighters again, taking medicine to sleep, eating poorly, and spending too much time sitting at a desk and staring at a computer screen. I gained weight and the fibroids grew.

Back to the retreat I went for another several weeks. It did the trick: I got my health, my joy, and my glow back; I shrank the fibroids again. Then I went back home, where the pendulum swung in the other direction. That became my cycle for the next few years.

What I was doing was delaying the inevitable. I wasn't making any of the difficult decisions that were facing me. My health continued to deteriorate. I was losing so much blood I developed anemia and had to receive iron infusions.

On one of my visits to the retreat, I bought a book at the shop on the campus: *Why People Don't Heal and How They Can* by Caroline Myss, a medical intuitive and bestselling author. When I read the following passage, it broke open something inside of me and for the first time in a long time, I was convinced that I had clarity.

"When an illness is a part of your spiritual journey, no medical intervention can heal you until your spirit has begun to make the changes that the illness was designed to inspire. Medical intervention, complementary healing modalities, changes in nutrition, and overall lifestyle may all help to some extent and should certainly be used. But the most effective healing option, when you are facing an illness as a spiritual challenge, is to rely on your spiritual practice to bring you the insights you need."

Between the sessions with Amy, my one and only Energy Healing session, the classes I'd taken at the retreat, as well as my own spiritual practice, which I'd been redefining and strengthening, I knew exactly what I had to do.

I called Dr. Woods and said, "Alright, let's do it. Let's schedule a time." I'd waited too long and had not dedicated my whole self to the naturopathic healing process. I was too sick, bleeding too heavily; my life was falling apart. I recognized that I needed to also heal from all the trauma I'd been carrying.

The morning of the procedure, I showed up at the medical facility wearing a stunning deep berry lip gloss and a sparkly tiara. I was in the process of making all the other changes I needed to make. I was writing my own work again, reclaiming my voice. Emotionally and spiritually, I felt solid. When I woke up in the post-op room, my daughter was sitting next to the bed.

"Mom," she said, as I searched the room to get my bearings. "You're awake now."

I smiled. "Yes. Please hand me my tiara and my lip gloss." I was ready to shine, to face my future. Little did I know that nearly everything in and about my life was about to come undone.

~

There is blood in my underwear. I see it while I am sitting on the toilet peeing. It's not a lot, about the same amount you see when you slice the pad of your thumb in the kitchen. That's hardly a comforting fact for a nine-year-old. Location matters. There are places where you shouldn't see blood, and inside your underwear is one of them. I think I'm dying, that the blood is leaking down from my heart or stomach. I don't know that blood from my stomach will not seep out through my vagina. I don't know anything about periods. I don't even know they exist. No one has explained any of this to me, yet. I don't know anything about my body.

My mother gives me a pad. It's like a brick made of layers and layers of napkins and cotton wool. It has two long flaps, one at the front and one at the back, that are supposed to be hooked onto a belt. My mother teaches me how to put it on, tie the belt. When we are done, I wear a new pair of underwear, pull my pants back up and walk awkwardly out of the bathroom. That is the extent of my education on menstruation.

It takes two years for me to bleed again. This time the flow is smooth, continuous, filling one pad after another, one day after another for four days. It is, by all measures, a standard period, complete with cramps. I still don't know the reason why I am bleeding, just that it is something women must do. No one explains that I am still a girl, yet parts of my body are making the transition to womanhood. No one explains how it is that my body can now produce another human being. The adults in my life tell me to be a good girl, to not do anything naughty with boys or else I'll get pregnant. What is good? What is naughty? Those two words, "good" and "naughty," are laced with blame, guilt, embarrassment, and shame—emotions that will follow me for the rest of my days.

Most of what I learn will come from school. Most will be rumors and old wives' tales. Some false, some true. I will believe them all until life teaches me otherwise. But why is life the one teaching me? Where are the women, the mothers and aunties who should be leading me through this rite of passage?

One year after that first for-real-for-real period, I am manipulated by a high school boy I have a crush on. He plays me like a fiddle, pretends he likes me too. He works hard to gain my trust, all the while knowing that he will soon break it. We kiss, we touch; I am curious, I am comfortable. Until I am not. But he doesn't stop, no matter how much I beg, or fight, or cry.

After him—days? weeks? I have made myself forget—it is a grown man. After that it is many young men.

Why does no one speak with me about consent? Why does no one teach me that with the reproductive organs I have, I wholly receive the energy of everyone who enters me. I receive their fears, their traumas, their rage, their love, and it either strengthens me or disrupts the harmony and flow of my body. This is the time to teach me that I am not a receptacle into which anything can be inserted.

Right now is when I need to learn to hold power in this body, to hold power in my voice, to exercise my right to say "no."

Right now is when the people in my life should encourage me to use the word "love" when I speak of my changing body and to look upon it with wonder and reverence.

As I move into menopause, I realize that this child on the cusp of puberty, this child that is still inside of me, is my guide. The road she is paving with the incidents in her life, with all the torment, defiance, and achievement, is the road that will lead her to where I now stand, holding every piece of the baggage she has accumulated.

—

After the surgery, my first symptoms were hot flashes and night sweats. I'd wake up and my pillowcase, bedsheet, and pajamas would be drenched. Dr. Woods had told me to expect this. Based on everything I'd ever heard—which, granted, was not much—menopause was pretty much defined by hot flashes, night sweats, the occasional headache, and vaginal dryness. But there is a plethora of other symptoms that nobody had ever mentioned to me. I didn't know that in addition to a hot flash—which feels as though there's a space heater in my body set on high—I could also experience a cold flush, a succession of arctic winds swirling around my ribcage, blowing through my heart's hollow chambers. Sometimes I felt as though I was on fire, other times it felt as though I'd been locked in a freezer.

One morning I discovered a long, spiky hair growing from the side of my mouth. Upon closer inspection, I realized there were more on each side. "I've started growing whiskers," I complained to Dr. Woods, "and I have hairs growing out of my neck." He assured me it was normal.

"Hormonal changes," he said, calmly.

"So, I'm just supposed to turn into the bearded lady?" He drew blood for tests to determine my hormone levels. That information, he said, would help him decide the best course of treatment. I told Dr. Woods I was also dealing with brain fog, weight gain, difficulty falling asleep, and depression. He advised that I try puzzles and other word games, the ketogenic diet, warm milk, and no devices an hour before bed. The depression, he believed, was a normal response to the surgery I'd just had. He felt it would lift sooner than later. This sounded plausible. I was no stranger to depression, but what I was contending with didn't feel at all like any of the episodes I'd had before, during which I'd been unable to get out of bed or leave the house. This time, I had difficulty concentrating. It was hard to read or watch television, and I was experiencing occasional suicidal ideation. I was sad and I was weepy, but otherwise functional.

Dr. Woods handed me a prescription and sample box of medication. I asked what it was for. "Vaginal dryness," he told me. Not once in that meeting had I mentioned the words "dry" and "vagina," either separately or together. I scrunched my lips, raised an eyebrow, and set the box on a stack of patient files on his desk.

"But I don't need this."

"I've been told it's a lifesaver. Your boyfriend will thank you for it." In the entire time that Dr. Woods and I had known each other, he'd never heard me speak of any man. Not a baby daddy, not a boyfriend, not a husband—each of which, at some point in our acquaintance, I'd had.

"I don't have a boyfriend."

"So, you're not sexually active?" I grabbed my purse and stood up. I was incensed. My body felt like a language in which I'd lost all fluency. I'd been hoping Dr. Woods could offer insight, if not actual help. Of all the maladies I'd mentioned, this man's priority was to make sure I didn't have a dry pussy— and he was doing it not for my sake, but to safeguard the sexual pleasure of another man, the one he believed I had in my life!

Eight or nine months following my surgery, the hot flashes and cold flushes stopped on their own. Around the same time, the depression abated, but I attributed that to psychiatry. I had a weekly talk therapy appointment with a psychiatrist who'd prescribed me an antidepressant, sleeping pills, and sedatives for anxiety. The sleeping pills and sedatives made me feel too groggy so I consulted a naturopath to see if there were herbal options. During our consultation, she told me that she didn't believe I was in menopause.

"You still have your ovaries. Every woman has a finite number of eggs. If you haven't released all of yours, then you're not in menopause." How then to explain the hot and cold flashes, the whiskers and brain fog?

"Those things can happen in perimenopause," she explained. "The partial hysterectomy was probably a shock to your body. It had to figure out how to continue functioning without the uterus. That most likely intensified symptoms of perimenopause that you were already having and brought on new ones."

"How will I know when I'm actually in menopause?" I asked. She suggested I use the age my mother entered menopause as an indication of when I might enter because without a uterus, there is no way to be certain. I'd been estranged from my mother for years. Even when we were not formally estranged, she'd never been a font of wisdom and sage advice in my life. I asked if there was any other way I could find out, and the answer was no.

There are tests that can be done to measure the levels of the follicle-stimulating hormone (FSH) that is produced in the pituitary gland and regulates the function of the ovaries. Consistently high FSH levels over a period of time are a strong indicator that a woman has reached menopause; however, during the transition from perimenopause to menopause, FSH levels can fluctuate wildly from day to day, so the only reliable indicator is the absence of a menstrual cycle for twelve contiguous months.

A year after the hysterectomy, I started experiencing even more symptoms. I was having issues with my balance and dizziness as well as with my memory. This was beyond brain fog. I couldn't remember people's names or words that I was about to use in a sentence. Even if I was able to fall asleep, staying asleep had become a problem. I would wake up at 4 a.m. every day and not be able to go back to sleep. I developed new allergies, and also started suffering from reflux and nausea. The depression returned and whereas the suicidal ideation had previously been sporadic, it was now continuous. I didn't know what was because of menopause and what wasn't. I didn't even know if I was really in menopause.

In allopathic medicine, the body is compartmentalized, divided into many supposedly disparate parts. In some instances, having physicians who specialize in one area of the anatomy may well be something to recommend, but it poses a significant problem for individuals going through menopause because its symptoms aren't centralized.

For every complaint, there was a doctor: an otolaryngologist, gastroenterologist, somnologist, neurologist, endocrinologist, psychiatrist, and, of course, gynecologist. At the time, not a single one of my doctors was Black or female. Each doctor wanted me to undergo comprehensive testing, so I spent many early mornings at the lab giving blood and urine, getting scans. They threw around names of possible illnesses, awful illnesses. They prescribed medicines whose list of possible side effects included such undesirable conditions as anal leakage, ruptured aorta, peeling of the skin in sheets. After a year or two of this, I thought for sure I was dying from some extremely rare degenerative disorder, and no one could tell me otherwise. Worse, no one could save me.

The turning point came when one of my doctors asked why I was taking a particular medication. It was the sedative my psychiatrist had prescribed for anxiety. The doctor informed me that multiple studies had shown the medicine causes accelerated cognitive decline. I was, yet again, incensed. In every single therapy session, I'd mentioned how worried I was about my brain blips and general fog. I'd mentioned my fear of dementia, ad nauseam; I'd explained that for a person who'd committed herself to a life of the mind, the loss of cognition, however gradual it may be, was terrifying. Why, then, would the psychiatrist prescribe a medication that would all but guarantee my worst nightmare? I went home, tossed all of my medications in the trash and canceled every upcoming doctor's appointment. Was anybody even listening to *me*, to *my* symptoms? Or were they just functioning by rote—ordering the requisite tests, prescribing the standard medication, operating from some medical script found in an old dusty reference book on human anatomy penned in the 1800s?

In the middle of yet another sleepless night, I returned to the book by Caroline Myss that I had, before my surgery, found extremely beneficial. I reread the section that had moved me to action: "When an illness is a part of your spiritual journey, no medical intervention can heal you until your spirit has begun to make the changes that the illness was designed to inspire."

My mind drifted to a seemingly unrelated subject. A common exercise in writing workshops is "a letter to your younger self." Now that you are older, presumably wiser, and have survived a few hardships of life, what would you want the younger version of yourself to know? I wondered if that exercise could work the other way around as well. What if your younger self could send you a message, something they wanted you to know, remember, or do when you got older? An informal time capsule.

I flashed to my past. Why had the sixteen-year-old me taken that pamphlet at the abortion clinic and hidden it in my pocket? Why, between then and now, had all the different versions of me felt compelled to keep it? It dawned on me that the cover of that pamphlet, which I now kept inside a clear plastic magnetized picture frame on my refrigerator door, could be a message from my younger self.

I walked into the kitchen, as if in a trance, stood in front of the fridge, and read aloud the words on the pamphlet's cover: *No woman is required to build the world by destroying herself.*

"Save yourself," my younger self seemed to be telling me. "Don't leave your fate in other people's hands."

At sixteen, I had not been able to save myself. I had been subjected to medical tests and procedures carried out by practitioners of questionable skill who did not consider or respect my wishes, let alone my body. They'd not had my best interest at heart. Granted, this wasn't the same situation; I wasn't being forced to terminate a pregnancy. Even so, I felt at the mercy of doctors who either did not listen, or refused to hear me.

It became clear that the only person who could heal me

was someone who knew and respected my history of survival; somebody who accepted and embraced my imperfect, aging body; somebody who did not think the color of my skin was an impediment or hindrance, someone who loved it. That person was me. Now I just had to figure out how to do it. I had to figure out how to save myself.

———

For every illness that exists, there is a flower, plant, tree, bush, shrub, fungi, or some tangled-up weed on the side of some dusty, rough road that will cure it. We are all capable of healing ourselves. People have been doing it since the beginning of time. And menopause is not a recent phenomenon.

My ailments were many, so I decided to begin by focusing on just one: sleep. Falling asleep, and staying asleep. I consulted a Traditional Chinese Medicine (TCM) practitioner, Dr. Chang, for a tongue and pulse diagnosis. He sent me home with a customized concoction of herbs. Before doing so, he spoke with me about sleep hygiene and offered a few suggestions. Those words of wisdom turned out to be of greater benefit than the herbs.

Dr. Chang wanted me to share with him the sleep routine I'd used for my daughter when she was a baby.

"You didn't let her watch television until just before she needed to sleep, did you?"

"No," I said.

"You didn't feed her a heavy meal and then straightaway put her in the crib, did you?"

"Of course not," I responded. His questions were ridiculous.

"Then why are you doing these things to yourself before you try to sleep?" I was speechless.

Dr. Chang advised me to set a regular bedtime and stop eating solid foods at least three hours before then; take a warm shower; wear pajamas or a nightgown instead of sweatpants and an old T-shirt; turn off the lights and all electronics that emit blue light; keep the room cool, almost a little chilly; and listen to an audiobook, soft music, or nature sounds. I decided to try this, and I quickly learned that it wasn't enough for me to want to be well, I had to be disciplined, mindful, and actively work to make these changes stick. It had to be my primary focus.

I rearranged my schedule, forced myself to turn off the computer, stop binge-watching television shows and doom scrolling on social media. Much to my surprise, I fell in love with audiobooks and the simple, exquisite pleasure of having someone tell you a story as you drift into slumber. And sleep always came, sometimes as quickly as five minutes from the time I started listening to the narration, but always within thirty minutes.

No matter what time I fell asleep, I would still wake up at 4 a.m. The audiobook would always help me get back to sleep, but I craved a night of deep, uninterrupted rest. I complained openly on social media, and one of my literary colleagues who was also going through menopause recommended using a weighted blanket. I quickly did some research, found out the correct weight that I needed, and bought one right away. The first night I used the blanket I did not wake up a single time.

Some nights, instead of an audiobook, I will listen to Yoga Nidra, a guided meditation that can be used to enter a fully relaxed state between sleep and consciousness.

Lack of sleep can have an adverse effect on memory and cognition. The better my sleep quality, the more improvement I noticed in my memory and brain fog. I continued doing crossword puzzles and other word challenges, as my former psychiatrist had suggested. I wrote by hand instead of with the computer. When a friend suggested learning new information was another way to exercise the brain and strengthen one's mental acuity, I started learning to speak Portuguese. Even with all that, I would still sometimes lose a word that had been on the tip of my tongue or blank out on an old friend's name. Whenever that happened, I would spiral into anxiety.

"Relax," another friend, who was postmenopausal, said. She pointed to her head and tapped an index finger against her temple. "Trust that it's in there. Stop and breathe, and give it a moment to rise to the surface. It happens to all of us, so don't be ashamed. Just say, 'I'm trying to find a specific word. It'll come to me,' and move on." And it always does come to me, sooner rather than later these days.

We humans are creatures of comfort. We resist change. We return and return to old habits until we finally adapt to a new routine. Every now and then, I would forget that my body no longer metabolized alcohol properly, or that I'd set a regular bedtime, or that I'd forbidden myself to eat several slices of pizza before bed. Sometimes what kept me up wouldn't be the food, alcohol, socializing, or television but grief, fear, or anxiety. After disrupting my sleep schedule, it would take as much as a week for me to get back into my routine. A younger friend who was in the midst of perimenopause urged me to go for a walk shortly after waking up. She'd also been having lots of problems with irregular sleep patterns and she swore by those morning walks. I heeded her advice and noticed that even if I'd stayed up later than I should to finish an assignment or attend an event, it now took little effort to go back to my regular routine.

"Do you know why that is?" my naturopath asked. She taught me that getting sunshine first thing in the morning resets the circadian rhythm by cueing the body to produce both serotonin and melatonin at the appropriate times to remain consistent with an individual's sleep schedule.

Walking is a gateway exercise. Once you start walking regularly, your body will crave even more movement. I tried yoga, Pilates, general stretching, and other exercises to improve my posture, my balance, and relieve my back pain and sciatica. I also exercise my pelvic floor.

Sleep and exercise were two of four significant pillars in my healing journey. The third was nutrition. I took vitamins, of course, but I decided to make it a point to get the bulk of my vitamins and minerals not from supplements but from my diet, by eating fresh whole, organic foods. I try not to eat out so that I have more control of what is and isn't in my foods. I also practice trophology, which is the science of food combining. Having attended the health retreat so often, I'd picked up a lot of useful information about various foods and their medicinal properties. Maca root, for instance, is an adaptogenic herb derived from an ancient Peruvian plant that I add into my daily smoothie. It balances hormones, relieves many symptoms of menopause, and improves libido. Every evening, I use a magnesium powder to prepare a warm pre-bedtime drink. I also use a magnesium-infused body butter to lotion myself after my evening shower. I make sure to rub it into the soles of my feet. It's a natural muscle relaxer, it lowers cortisol levels, and it improves sleep. And I drink loads of water, stopping a couple of hours before I go to bed to ensure I am able to sleep through the night. Changing the way that I ate changed the way I felt pretty much immediately. It is almost criminal that in our medical system, nutrition is an afterthought, if even that.

The fourth and final pillar in my healing journey has been joy. I'm writing, reading, building a social life, doing the things I love. Life was so heavy for so long; it felt like if I lowered my arms, let them rest, the sky would come crashing down. But how many times can the same sky fall?

You know, in the United States, unless we belong to certain indigenous tribes or religions, there are no formal rites of passage. We enter the most defining parts of our lives, the ones that serve as transitions from one stage to another, without fanfare, spiritual recognition, or ritual. Instead of celebration, each stage is characterized by secrecy, misinformation, and fear. And none more than menopause because it also means growing old, and our society does not permit women to grow old.

What I realized when I entered menopause and finally learned to navigate and love this new body is that I am free. It is, perhaps, the first time in my life I have felt so wholly unencumbered, unfazed, just free. Far from being invisible, I am able to see myself truly, without the silly masks of politeness, and false humility that society imposes on young women. Fuck what anybody thinks. I have a right to be here. I have a right to speak, to shout, to moan, to purr, to curl myself into the tight corners of joy as surely as I have been wound into spaces of sorrow.

When I was younger, I was moved by a poem titled "Warning," by Jenny Joseph, an excerpt of which reads:

> When I am an old woman I shall wear purple
> With a red hat which doesn't go, and doesn't suit me.
> […] I shall go out in my slippers in the rain
> And pick flowers in other people's gardens
> And learn to spit.

Back then, I didn't understand the poem. Of course, I knew what it meant literally. I loved the imagery. What I didn't get, though, was the joy; I didn't see the absolute pleasure of flouting society's norms and mores to be one's own quirky self. Not being so worried about what everyone says or thinks, not trying to be "good" or "smart" or "nice" or any of the words that are taped onto the mouths of girls and women to silence them so they can't speak their minds, or learn to love the sound of their own voices.

Back then, I didn't identify with anything beyond the words "old woman," because I'd been taught to fear both age and womanhood. I read that poem and all I saw was lunacy. Since then, I have come to understand that sometimes liberation can look like that. Joy can look like that.

RIDE

By Gina Frangello

Nature didn't intend for women to be sexually active after menopause…
—*Harvard Health Publishing (2021)*

Let me take you on a ride, the way my body has been on a ride. By the time you are holding this book in your hands, it will have been a decade at least since I first got strapped in and found myself, for many years, unable to get off what seemed a deranged roller coaster, with its constant pitching downward and centrifugal force that held me in place when the world was upside down. Let me take you on a ride that seemed, for the longest of times, as though all I would ever be able to do was hold on and try to keep from throwing up all over myself. Like all rides, this one begins with a thrill, a rush of adrenaline, before things take a terrifying turn, before I came to believe that the ride would never end: that this was My Life Now. Come with me back to late November, 2015, when I am already queued up for this ride but don't know it yet.

It starts something like this:

You can do anything you want to me.

I am forty-seven years old, and this is my favorite line when my partner, Rob, and I have sex. We whisper, moan, rapturously breathe into each other's mouths. Sometimes, I half-sob it ecstatically, back arched as he clutches my hair in his fist while he fucks me from behind, yanking me into a near backbend so he can slap my face. We write this phrase back and forth in frantic emails, describing what we will do to each other the next time we can be together in person. He first purred it at me more than three years ago, when I burned him with a violet wand until his skin shot sparks. Unconditional mutual surrender is our aphrodisiac.

There are words in the BDSM community for what we do— what we are. *Switches. Respecting and expanding boundaries.* But these terms feel generic and clinical, and I am a Midwestern mom of three who doesn't run in kink circles anyway. My every desire feels specific to *this man*, to the alchemy between us. Although I was married for twenty-two years, had a varied and complex life that included both decades of marital sex and the shorter relationships, flings, and one-night stands that preceded my marriage at twenty-five, I often feel like I barely comprehended what sex even was before Rob. *I love you like we invented it*, we used to sign our emails. We are both middle-aged, cognizant that our reaction to each other might look over-blown, melodramatic, to many of our friends. We say *I love you* twenty times a day. We can rarely be near each other without touching, fall asleep holding, sucking, clutching each other's bodies. Bottomless desire moves in me like a gravitational force constantly catapulting my stomach down an elevator shaft, my skin buzzing electric. *More, more, more.*

Rob and I started as a casual literary connection when I published a story of his in 1998, then blossomed slowly—gloriously, treacherously—over the next dozen years into an intimate friendship that in early 2012 exploded into an extra-marital affair and finally ruptured our respective troubled marriages in April 2015.

Finally, we are free to be together. There are logistical and emotional hurdles galore. We live two thousand miles apart; my children are dealing with the fallout of my divorce—in no way ready for a man they barely know to move into our home—and Rob can't afford steep LA rents in addition to costly travel every few weeks to Chicago to see me, so he is still crashing in his ex's apartment. Nevertheless I find myself smiling uncontrollably whenever I drive alone in my car. I am forty-seven years old. My life feels new; I have never felt so beautiful or alive.

Then, one night during sex, my shimmering new life barely off the ground, I have, unbeknownst to me at the time, reached the front of the line and am about to board my Years-Long Ride: Rob feels a lump in my left breast.

I have always been just slightly ahead of my mother's curve. I got married four years younger than she did, became a mother three years earlier, and in keeping with this tradition, I go into menopause three years earlier than she did, when I am still forty-seven, in my first month of chemotherapy for breast cancer.

My mother claimed she "barely noticed" menopause. "I just stopped getting my period," she told me. "I never had hot flashes or any of those things." She never went on hormone therapy, despite it being nearly ubiquitous in 1982 when my mother, at the age of fifty, stopped bleeding.

At the time of my mother's "change of life," she was in a platonic marriage with my father—they had not made love since the year I was conceived. She was a stay-at-home mother who had not yet returned to the workforce, which she would do the following year when my father's medical bills for his perpetually bleeding ulcer catapulted us from "regular poor" to being so in need of economic triage that a job in the windowless basement of a preschool, paying $9,000 annually, seemed like a gift from heaven.

As a younger woman, my mother had looked like Isabella

Rossellini—she had sung in smoky jazz bars—yet by the age of fifty she had taken to wearing shapeless knockoffs of Laura Ashley dresses and matching tops and bottoms that reminded me of Garanimals. I loved my mother more than anyone else on earth.

It was also my entire mission in life to grow up to be nothing like her.

One moment, my cycle was as regular as if I were still twenty-five; I was having the hottest sex of my life. Then, within a matter of months, both my breasts are gone, scraped down to the bone; I've lost my hair (everywhere); I will never have a period again. Besides the ordeal of cancer, I am also in the midst of a high-conflict divorce and have just lost both my father and my job.

For the first time in my life, my mother's experience comes back to me as an inspirational road map rather than an aversion. "Menopause," I often quip, channeling her stoicism, "is the least of my worries."

"I have some hot flashes," I tell friends dismissively, "but it's probably just the chemo."

Move along, people, nothing to see here.

Or rather, there is so much to see that my lost blood had better be the least of the spectacle.

Meanwhile, my journalistic background, history in academia, and writerly curiosity get the better of me—on the sly and against my own desire to even *know*, I begin doing what I always do: research deep diving. Most of what I read strikes me as more bleak than if I discovered my hair would never grow back.

A 2010 Journal of Sexual Medicine study reports that 70 percent of women diagnosed with breast cancer face issues with sexual functioning two years later.

*After menopause, libido declines, and changes in our bodies can make it difficult to get aroused, painful to have intercourse, and impossible to climax. It's little wonder that many women become dissatisfied with sex, and some avoid intimacy entirely.**

According to Kelly Connell on Caring.com, chemo in particular can "wreak havoc on a woman's ability to orgasm."

Without ever quite making a conscious decision, I grow determined to be the exception to every statistic, to prove the disturbing status quo wrong.

In 2016, Rob and I wait in pre-op before my breast reconstruction surgery. I'm in a hospital gown, but I can still feel the expander—blown up with saline—where my breasts used to be. The expander was installed during my mastectomy and feels like a metallic tube top that I constantly want to reach down and untangle but can't because it is under my skin. I'm considerably less excited to "have breasts again" than I am to just get this fucking expander out of my body.

---

* "Yes, You Can Have Better Sex in Midlife and in the Years Beyond," Harvard Health Publishing, Harvard Medical School, September 30, 2021, https://www.health.harvard.edu/womens-health/yes-you-can-have-better-sex-in-midlife-and-in-the-years-beyond.

Outside, it's June, but here, being wheeled into yet another operating theater in a hospital that is starting to feel entirely too much like home, it could be any season, any year—here, time stands still. Finally, this is the surgery that is supposed to get me Out of Here, so bring it on! I try to remember when I last *felt unequivocally good* in my body, but although I'd like to tell myself it was the night before my mastectomy, when Rob and I last had sex with my Former Body, in truth that was the most depressing fuck of my life—the only time I've ever suspected I was the target of a pity fuck. It didn't help when Rob abruptly stopped after making me come and declined to climax himself.

When I get out of surgery this time, my new breasts are bandaged up, so it isn't until we get home that I can stand in front of a mirror and survey them bare. I'm in so much shock I can hardly process my own image. Who *is* that, looking back at me, bruised, stubble-headed, and…with enormous tits? Rob and I both stare at them, not saying anything, digesting in confusion what has occurred. Precancer, I was an A cup. I have told my plastic surgeon some 850 times that, for my reconstruction, I would like to be "a perfect B." These things inside my body are *definitely* not a B.

I will find out later, when I go to get measured for new bras, that my new breasts are, in fact, Ds. But here, standing in what has become a fun-house, distorted mirror, I feel like someone removed Pamela Anderson's nipples and stapled her remaining breasts onto my body. They torpedo out like a shelf; I could hang things from them. There is no organic breast tissue left in my body, so there's no gradated swelling like real cleavage—they shoot straight out from my chest wall. I stand there saying, "Ohmygod ohmygod," until I sink my head into my hands and collapse on the bed.

Rob sits next to me, rubbing circles on my back. "You'll get used to them," he says, clearly trying to make me feel better.

"You're from LA!" I practically scream. "People there do this crazy shit on purpose!"

When we go back to the plastic surgeon (who came highly recommended, who loves poetry, who wears a bow tie), he shrugs and says something like, "You're very petite. In my experience, when you give a petite woman a smaller cup size, the implants look too wide and flat for her frame, like pectoral muscles. These are teardrop shaped, the most realistic model. They look more natural sized up."

(At this point, having been informed that my male surgeon basically decided to give me porn star tits without consulting me because he was *afraid I might look like a man*, I have a cardiac arrest, drop dead in his office, and am no longer alive to be writing this essay... sorry.)

But, of course, having been raised female, having been raised to make everyone comfortable, having spent the last year of my life both terrified of my litigious ex-husband *and* listening to my divorce attorney worry aloud that my "boyfriend" is going to leave me for getting cancer, what I actually do is sit meekly on the examining table while the plastic surgeon uses a syringe to extract bits of fat from other parts of my body to inject into the tops of my Torpedo Tits, to create a more natural décolletage.

Admittedly, it works, and my breasts no longer look like cyborg porn anime, though they are still—to me—enormous.

*   *   *

It's October 2016, and Rob and I are in Los Angeles staying in his best friend's guest room, and we are trying to be quiet. Rob's belt is fastened around my arms and torso tightly while he goes down on me, and my left arm feels weird. The belt is well below my new breasts, which still feel like tennis balls sewn into my chest, but something is wrong. I flew to LAX only hours ago, not wearing a compression garment on my left arm because nobody on my medical team has ever indicated that I *should* do that, or even told me that such garments exist or where I can obtain them, much less that flying—which I have done almost a dozen times since my mastectomy—is a trigger for lymphedema. I know vaguely what lymphedema is, but my oncology team mentioned it only in passing, saying to be careful about lifting heavy objects with my left arm but that my risk is low because I'm "young and thin."

I have not thought of lymphedema since that brief exchange, but I remember it now, a strange heaviness in my left arm that I don't recognize, as though sluggish, acidic liquid is moving too slowly just under my skin. Obviously, no one on my oncology team has given me any tips on post-mastectomy bondage—in fact, they have not mentioned sex at all other than having given me a handbook that I threw in the recycling bin the moment I read that I might never orgasm again post-chemo. I *can* still orgasm, so that book can fuck off. Rob and I started having sex again less than a week after my mastectomy, and I have wasted no time broadcasting that news to my doctor, my therapist, my friends. *Look, I'm still me!*

It's hard to focus on my clit right now, which no longer contains the hypersensitivity I've known since my first orgasm. Truth be told, my clit is a little numb, has a long on-ramp these days, and this sluggish, syrupy arm pain is taking precedence. I don't say that aloud, though, because if I do, Rob will undo the belt, will fuss and cluck over me with worry, and the thought of it all makes my skin crawl. What happened to *You can do anything you want to me?* I hold my tongue, close my eyes, scroll through some of my trusty fantasies (that don't involve not being able to make a sound while in a friend's guest room), and eventually my brain outwits my arm and I twist around the bed in climax—*fuck you, ten-pound cancer handbook I threw away.*

Even after Rob unties me, I don't mention anything about my misbehaving left arm.

Fake it till you make it, my friend Kathy used to say, until she died of complications from ovarian cancer in 2011. But I don't *have* to fake it, I reassure myself. If I no longer have an A+ in Orgasms, I still have a solid B.

A few days later, I board the roughly four-hour flight home, still without the compression garment I don't know exists. On my left wrist, I wear a cuff bracelet I got in Kenya six years ago, and as I stand at baggage claim waiting for my luggage, I notice that I feel sweaty under the cuff, that it feels tighter than usual even though the Velcro only fastens in one way, and it is always the same size. I absentmindedly glance down at my bracelet to see if something is wrong with it.

That's when I notice that my wrist is about 25 percent larger than its normal size, swollen and puffy, straining against the Velcro the way I failed to struggle against my restraints back in the LA guest room. *More more more.* I stare down at my wrist. When my mother's best friend had breast cancer, her entire arm swelled to the size of a thigh, I abruptly recall—she had to wear a brace-like garment on it 24/7 to prevent it getting bigger still.

I have cried exactly once since my cancer diagnosis: on the morning of my mastectomy, before going to the hospital, when I sobbed into Rob's chest that I'd ruined everybody's life—his, my children's—by leaving my long marriage and then inconveniently getting cancer like some grotesque bait and switch, and that maybe everyone would be better off if I just died.

Now I cry for the second time, staring down at my sweating, swollen wrist, the marks from the cuff imprinted into my lymph-logged skin. Nobody even looks my way. Airports are overrun with crying people; my tears are cheap.

Sometimes, the ride slows down for a while, enough that I can ooh and ahh at the surprisingly magnificent views. Sometimes, it feels like the ride has stopped entirely, and I'm off now, back on solid ground. Sometimes, so many crises have been averted (*I'm not dead! I didn't lose custody of my children! I've found new work!*) that I feel like the whole purpose of the ride was to make me grateful every minute of every day. Sometimes I worry that if I forget, even momentarily, to bask in gratitude, the ride will start up again to punish me. Sometimes, though, I forget to torture myself with these superstitions and I am actually happy, not so much "again" as in a new way, an uncharted waters kind of wild happiness I've never previously known.

Defying my divorce attorney's (and no doubt plenty of other people's) predictions, Rob moves to Chicago full-time near the end of 2017, bringing with him a slew of guitars, amps, books, and exactly two pieces of beat-up furniture. For the first time ever, we get to fall asleep together every night and wake up together in the morning. He loves to bring me coffee in bed, and in the evenings, we rejoice that our master bedroom is upstairs, distanced from the three kids', given we have sex nearly every night. I am forty-nine years old. Many nights, Rob and I hold each other, whispering back and forth, "Who *gets* this? Who gets to *have* this?" and, giddy, kissing, out of our heads with relief and love, murmur into each other's mouths, "We're so lucky. Us. *We* do."

If anyone were to walk up to me with a clipboard and ask whether being catapulted into instant menopause—much less anything related to my cancer—caused me to experience "sexual dysfunction," the term most often used in studies and articles, I would still give an immediate and emphatic no. I would not consider this a lie. I am having more sex than I've ever had in my life, with a partner to whom my attraction feels all-consuming and singular. I am orgasming, even if no longer as speedily as a rocket, and in our consumer capitalist culture, where even sex is often equated with orgasm as "product," I am still decidedly "productive."

I am not like the poor women in those studies. I am nothing, nothing like my mother.

One thing about this ride: Sometimes, it speeds along two tracks at once. It can't always just pick a direction and stay there. The ride contains more than one Truth.

What I would not admit to any aforementioned, hypothetical clipboard-wielding researcher, much less to my friends or the man with whom I share a bed:

1. Whereas I had regularly masturbated since college, hitting a peak of frequency in the Affair Years of 2012–2015 when Rob and I sometimes went as long as four or five months without seeing each other, I have now stopped masturbating almost entirely, even when he is out of town.

2. I have longed my entire life for a man to whom I can not only confess my every desire without embarrassment but with whom I can be assured those desires will be enthusiastically fulfilled. Yet even though I now have precisely that emotional and sexual trust in my partner, I have lost

all desire to be spanked, bound, slapped, bitten, etc., or even fucked roughly.

Rob and I originated as friends and confidants, progressed to co-conspirators and partners in crime, and throughout all that time I was ruthlessly and radically honest with him about my every thought and action. Now here we are, a Real Couple, no need to hide in the shadows, no need for lies. And yet I find myself incapable of articulating that the walls of my vagina feel inflamed and sore every time he enters me either missionary style or from behind, or that when he rests too much of his body weight on me or flips me on my stomach, I harbor an intense fear that my weirdly large breasts will explode. Also, the eradication and rebuilding of my immune system during chemo seems to have accelerated my previously mild osteoarthritis such that my left hip is now bone-on-bone, full of bone spurs and cysts. Between that and the aromatase inhibitor I'm on that squelches any residual postmenopausal estrogen straight out of my body (to keep it from feeding further breast cancer), if Rob makes even the slightest attempt to spank me, it feels like he has plugged my hip directly into an electric socket—not in a hot way.

And so, in the months between my cancer and his Chicago move, our sex life has slowly tilted toward my taking a dominant role with ever-increasing frequency. Before my cancer/menopause, we had a highly fluid dynamic that—when power exchanges were included—probably skewed 60/40 toward my being in the submissive role, and we also had plenty of intense, transcendent, so-called vanilla sex. These days, though, I crave control. While Rob was always fascinatingly creative in coming up with things to do to me (I used to joke that he planned sex like other people plan vacations), abruptly I find myself taking charge of every sexual encounter before he can act on any of his ideas that might not "work" for my new, precarious body. My sexual personality has changed so entirely that it must seem I'm secretly taking Domme classes while he sleeps...even when we're just fucking, I always want to be on top to control the pace and depth of penetration.

If Rob is confused by my sudden hunger to be the one calling the shots, he certainly isn't complaining. In fact, at this particular aspect of the ride, he seems enthralled.

Have you heard the one about men's desire being for the woman, but the woman's desire being for the desire of the man?

The more excited Rob is by my taking charge...well, the more charge I take. Soon, I barely remember our old effortless fluidity when we so organically swapped roles, positions, vibes. I barely recall the way *anything* seemed possible, our private island of sex spread out like uncharted territory.

Now, *I* am the carnival conductor of our sex life, pulling levers to direct our ride this way or that. By day, I go to doctor appointments, to oncologists and physical therapists and orthopedic surgeons. I get cortisone shots to soothe my hip, drink Chinese powdered herbs, pop Duexis and tramadol like M&M'S

---

* The full version of this quote is attributed to Samuel Taylor Coleridge.

so that I can fucking walk. Anesthetized by pain meds, joint-achy and hormonally neutered by anastrozole, it takes longer and longer to climax, so increasingly I choose activities not involving my orgasm.

It's a common adage that many men enjoy being submissive because they're in positions of power all day and it feels good to abandon control. If that theory is true, then I've become a case study in the inverse, trying through sexual dominance not to seem weak, lost, prematurely aged and hopelessly altered, a stranger to myself. Whereas I was once a spontaneity junkie who loved not knowing where the night would lead, now I fear the unexpected, work overtime to keep my lover so entertained that he will never feel compelled to suddenly switch up the scene.

Finally, it works so well that he mainly stops trying.

Um…mission accomplished?

"A Victorian woman going through the menopause was often considered to be emotionally unstable. During this 'climacteric period', she may well have been prescribed leeching or bloodletting from the ankle. Her doctor would have advised against reading novels, going to parties and dancing. For a 45–50 year old Victorian woman, an onslaught of instability and madness was considered inevitable."*

---

* "The Wandering Womb," RCN Women's Health Forum, the History of Nursing Society and Library and Archive Service, www.rcn.org.uk /library-exhibitions/Womens-health-wandering-womb.

*   *   *

It is early 2018, and I am at the Pain Clinic, where I've been coming for some months. My hip has disintegrated such that I have only a few inches range of movement in any direction and am in constant chronic pain that sends sharp jolts through my groin when I walk and radiates downward all the way from the outer side of my leg to my ankle when I am sitting or lying down. I have just urinated into a cup for drug testing, because to be prescribed pain medication here, you must test negative for any other kind of drug, even CBD (which I'd like to take for my pain but had to stop because it can show up as THC).

My Pain Clinic doctor is about my age, and sometimes he is chatty and a bit flirtatious with me, but today he has a younger resident with him and is all business. I am here to make a case— here with my drugless urine; here with my chemo-gnawed hip, my left leg so weak that I have to ascend stairs on my ass and hoist my leg with my hands to get into my SUV. I am here today on a mission and my desire is simple: I want to be taken off tramadol and given a higher or more frequent dose of Norco, because the tramadol, I explain to these two men—one young enough to be my son—makes it virtually impossible for me to orgasm.

"I looked it up." Being a researcher, I am also *that patient* who never adheres to doctors' advice to stay off the internet. "Tramadol is sometimes used for men who have premature ejaculation."

The resident mutters something about never having heard about tramadol being used that way. I don't tell him that I gave a couple of pills to a friend of mine whose husband always comes too soon and that she called it a godsend and is at this moment trying to figure out how to get a prescription. I stay quiet and nonthreatening. Being nonthreatening is important at the Pain Clinic, where there is always some out-of-control man screaming at the receptionist—where people lose their shit when they can't get as many pills as they want. I am 5'1", a nearly fifty-year-old cancer survivor and mother of three; my urine cup is all good, nothing threatening about me. I explain, "Sometimes, the tramadol makes me take a *really* long time, where it's kind of Project Orgasm, and other times, I can't climax at all."

The doctor who sometimes flirts with me smiles, makes eye contact, and something in me relaxes. Maybe all I had to do was ask.

Then he says to me, with utter seriousness despite the smile on his face, "Well, are your orgasms really that important?"

My mother died abruptly, upright in her recliner with the television remote control still in her hand and absolutely zero sign that, even in her final moments, she had found anything out of the ordinary about the day.

Sometimes I hear her in my head saying, *Dying was so easy, I hardly noticed it.*

If you're on any ride long enough, one thing you will inevitably learn is that, like some recurring dream, it turns out you've been on this ride many times before and just didn't know it. Some-times, the ride comes with a pair of goggles you didn't notice at first, through which you can finally see in the dark.

Growing up, it was my job to be easy. My mother was like an alien in our neighborhood, where all the other mothers of young children were more than a decade younger than she was, and where my father's favorite brother called her "The Hill-billy" (because if she wasn't Italian, Puerto Rican, Jewish, or Black, what else *was* there?). Although no one ever couched it in these terms at the time, she suffered from longstanding clinical depression over her marriage to a man who managed to be inde-pendent to the point of inconsideration (we would often walk into a room to find my father had left the house without telling anyone)—and yet needed her for every minute task from mak-ing doctors' appointments to managing the checkbook.

My mother possessed an innate optimism at odds with her narrow life—she was the type to grasp at any straws of happiness—and so she lived vicariously through me, her "mir-acle baby." I was the daughter everyone said she could never conceive due to her polycystic ovarian syndrome, the baby her obstetrician said would likely be born dead due to her advanced maternal age (thirty-five) and gestational diabetes. For as long as I could remember, I had been her entire world: her only source of joy, her symbiotic confidante. She called me her "best friend," which made me uncomfortable in ways I couldn't articulate.

During my youth, my mother experienced me as porous: Everything I carried leaked in under her own skin. If I came home in turmoil about some seventh-grade friendship drama or seemed down and insecure because a high school crush didn't like me back, my mother's face would deflate. She would magnify my problems as if under a spotlight, asking about them constantly. I took this on: understood I must not say or do anything to elicit these reactions of her distress. Maybe I was born allergic to pity.

By the age of eleven, I had started performing for her benefit. In this version of my life, told over the kitchen table after school or while lying around my mother's bedroom together, I was endlessly tough, swaggering, sought after, indestructible. My mother could not overreact to my miseries because they didn't exist: This version of Me had no problems. On the rare occasions that I could not conceal my issues from her, the price was steep. Once, when I was suffering from panic attacks and anorexia in the aftermath of college graduation, she told me that my "emotional distance" had "damaged our relationship permanently." Though this did not turn out to be true, it remains one of the most painful things anyone has ever said to me.

I learned to comfort my mother whenever she was sad, to keep her confidences about my father or her family of origin (that I often did not wish to hear), to perpetually entertain her so as to keep the noonday demon of her claustrophobic circumstances at bay. Now, I know pop psychology phrases that can reduce our relationship to labels, but they sell short how boundlessly I loved her.

I resist the notion that we are all defined by the worst of ourselves.

Still, every day after school, from the time I was in sixth grade, I was my mother's Scheherazade, saving myself from her reactions had she known how profoundly unhappy I really was, and saving *her* from having to look her own life in the face. My mother made me a storyteller, and I spent decades of my life unspooling an extremely long autofiction for her, hiding so many parts of myself from view that I could no longer even discern what might be called my "real self."

To be easy is a skill, and being an easy daughter was a thing I had been honing for more than a decade by the time I met my first husband and set out upon my attempts to be an easy wife, an endeavor I believed successful until it wasn't. Still, when he and I had troubles—which we often did—I held them close to my chest in public so that everyone around us, my mother included, believed me flawlessly happy. Some thought me stupidly oblivious to the problematic dynamics in my marriage, others took my performance for fact, expressing envy at my "perfect life."

When I left that life behind, I was supposed to be embracing a new period of authenticity. I was supposed to be rejecting the patriarchal notions that a middle-aged mother's sole purpose is to make her husband and children comfortable. Choosing a life with Rob meant leaping off a cliff of radical belief: a belief that my own desires and feelings actually *counted* for something. Yet here I was again, in some twisted full circle, performing for Rob even though he'd said for years that he didn't expect or want that.

Did he notice that I no longer obsessively regaled him with my every outlandish sexual fantasy? Terrifyingly, I found myself rarely thinking about sex except when we were in the midst of having it. Did this just seem normal now that we lived in the same house and could have sex any time we wanted? Did measuring my sexual satisfaction by how easily I climaxed even make *sense*, when I had reliably orgasmed in my first marriage and yet had always felt deeply sexually lonely?

My stomach still pitched and leaped whenever Rob and I had intense conversations, when I read his writing, when I watched him play guitar, or when his eyes glowed as I entered a room...but to whom was I supposed to explain that although I was still deeply *attracted to* my partner, that no longer translated to getting instantly wet, no longer made my body vibrate internally, longing for wild release? Wouldn't I just be told that relationships were "like that"—that time tamped down feral desire? Or, more likely, wouldn't any doctor, therapist, friend, just smile indulgently at me as though I was a fool not to fall to my knees in gratitude that my hot partner even wanted to fuck my nippleless, limping body at all?

In fact, my partner seemed rather rapturous about my scarred up, limping body. I also knew—from reading, from talking to other women—that some breast cancer survivors feel trauma or embarrassment at having their chests looked at or touched. Yet although I did not feel *ashamed* of my new body, I still felt like I was wearing a costume.

*   *   *

After two years of trying every possible remedy for my chronic pain, I finally succumbed to a hip replacement the month before my fiftieth birthday. Given the events of the years leading up to this, nobody could possibly accuse my life of being perfect anymore. There was no illusion to protect. Yet somehow, I was still on the stage, performing my perpetual "okayness" in the bedroom, terrified of ending up desexualized like my mother had been. Had it really taken me two years to realize that this was a barrier not only to Rob's and my otherwise full-throttle intimacy, but to my actual experience of spontaneous desire? Somehow, I had fallen back into an old trap of believing my in-the-moment, vulnerable self was not enough... only this time, in this relationship, I understood that fear was entirely on me.

You can take the woman out of the one-woman show, but it's infinitely harder to take the one-woman show out of the woman.

One month after my hip replacement, Rob and I get engaged. Between menopausal weight gain that wasn't helped by two years of pain and disability, and my larger breasts, most of my favorite clothes no longer fit me, but little by little I push myself to get back into yoga and Pilates, learning the true north of my new body. My size 2 dresses will never again zip up over these breasts, and my postmenopausal stomach will never again be perfectly flat, but by now I've gained the perspective to understand that these truths impact my quality of life not at all.

That summer of 2018, what I often think instead is that I would gladly gain thirty *more* pounds if it somehow magically meant I'd get my old libido back. But like my original breasts, like my left hip's cartilage, those old desires feel impossible to recapture.

Accept it, I tell myself. I've been telling myself a story about how all the statistics about postmenopausal, post-cancer sexuality have nothing to do with me based on how *often* I have sex, on how sexy I still find my partner, on everything except my own feelings…but it is time to accept that these statistics are my story, too—that I am not an "exception." And that maybe, no one ever said I had to be.

"The only constant in life is change" is a saying credited to the Greek philosopher Heraclitus. And so it is, surprisingly, slowly, as I move my body more, with radically less pain—as my body adjusts to the changes of menopause, to its cyborg reinvention—that the ride begins to shift again.

Rob, it turns out, however much he has been enjoying my forays into unexpected levels of sexual dominance, begins to lose some of the trepidation he clearly felt about my Body in Pain, and sometimes, when I am least expecting it, he begins to mix things up again. I discover that if I wear my lymphedema garment, I can still be bound—discover that, now that my left hip is not a raw exposed nerve, the sweet spot on my ass that used to so hum with ecstasy when he spanked/cropped/caned it is safe to touch again.

One night he surprises me with a massage table as a gift and soon begins massaging me a couple nights a week when I get home from work. Sometimes, his hands are therapeutic—the breaking up of scar tissue; slow but determined deep work on my IT bands—but even when it hurts, I find the self that had been in perpetual performance mode going dormant. My body is learning again to *just feel*, to lean in until I am in a languid trance almost similar to so-called sub space, even though, technically, he is the one "serving" me.

No longer on prescription painkillers since my successful hip replacement, my orgasms stop feeling like homework and, alleviated of my constant fear that Project Orgasm won't *work*, I begin to deeply crave coming again, even if not with the daily frequency of my premenopausal days, even if it takes a bit longer than it used to. Most surprisingly of all, in the absence of my nipples—which used to feel like a direct line to my clit— my vaginal opening grows more sensitive and if it and my clit are stimulated at the same time, I come with an intense ferocity I've never experienced, my body bucking into a V-shape, up and down, several times as I ride the waves.

One day, at our little cabin in the California desert, when Rob is spanking me, I also find myself doing something I always nurtured fantasies about but never achieved: openly sobbing. Maybe, after everything my body has been through, I've somehow *let go* enough to make it possible. The tears feel like a pent-up dam—like the pressure of the last seven years of my life flowing out of me like toxins—and frantically I grab for my red vibrator, ordering Rob, "Harder, yes, more," the whoosh of the cane in my ears when I climax thunderously.

For whatever reason, it stills and soothes something in me, puts me more fully in the present moment than even meditation, and I come out of my trance feeling cleansed, euphoric...not that dissimilarly to the way I feel after an hours-long massage, actually, though on the face of things, these two acts have little in common.

It turns out, there are many, many rides in this particular amusement park. It turns out, I'm not trapped after all. All I have to do is unfasten my seatbelt and get out.

Once upon a time, my mother was a singer, but it was only after her death, when I was fifty, that I, too, began to sing. Five years later, Rob's and my band has played street festivals, Joni Mitchell tributes, and double sets around Chicago, my voice rasp-screaming into the mic in a way the old version of me, who kept everything so close to her chest and never dared look foolish, would never have allowed. With all the confused longing of a recovering Catholic atheist daughter of a lapsed Protestant, and despite every mistake we each made along the way, I hope my mother can somehow hear me, and know my voice would not exist without hers.

Rob has moved his red lava lamp up from his basement office into our bedroom, where we practice and record, because he insists, every studio needs a lava lamp. Sometimes at night, when we are having whatever kind of sex we want to be having that night, the lava lamp gives the room a red glow, and we laugh about how the small windows in our attic room must be emanating a red light out onto the street like our bedroom is Amsterdam. In the Amsterdam of our imagination, even if *You can do anything you want to me* no longer applies in quite the same way, it is still gloriously true that *anything we damn well want* goes.

And what do women—and all menstruating and post-menstrual human beings—want? We want not to be a one-dimensional fictional monolith. We want to be recognized as fully human, to be seen and heard, to embody our mortal coils without having to perform femininity, prepackaged sexiness, low-maintenance, and flawless strength for others. We want the right to be individuals, with all our quirks and kinks and hopes and fears, without being expected to go quietly into the night of "quaintness" just because we are older than we once were.

Rob and I do not go back to the submission/dominance ratios of our old sex life before my body's changes…maybe in part because what constitutes submission and dominance itself feels more complicated and intertwined now? On the massage table—which would, in the general public, not even be considered "sex" per se—Rob is in the role of the giver, but he is also the active one, exercising a certain amount of control over my body, in which, like when one sexually submits, I don't have to think, act, make any decisions, and am just in a form of pure being, whether the sensations are gentle, erotic, painful, intense. Besides, now that I'm not stuck in some vortex of needing to perform strength, I'm able to see that Rob's sexual tastes and desires are evolving too . . . I'm not the only one who hasn't stood still, set in stone as some former version of myself. And so, slowly, we begin to talk more openly about the ways in which my physical changes impacted what I felt safe wanting, and he begins to open up more fully to me, too, about things he was previously self-conscious to ask for.

If familiarity is the death of desire, *genuine intimacy* is the ultimate aphrodisiac.

In the summer of 2019, my twin daughters and I bring some of my mother's ashes to Banff and scatter them in Lake Louise, where she always longed to go. There, we spend a grueling, magical day hiking up to a tea house where a European couple buys us tuna salad sandwiches and shares their table. We look out over the white-haired mountains that stand sentry above the lake, and I feel overcome with grief and regret that, during the last years of my mother's life, my head was so far up my own ass—between my affair, my divorce, my cancer, my scrambling to make a living, my years of chronic pain—that I never made the time to take her here myself. It's time I'll never get back, a thing I have to live with going forward. My mother is gone, and all the years I spent trying not to become her feel muddled and misguided in retrospect. How repulsed I felt, at times, by her body, blaming her for her weight gain and neediness with my father. Maybe those demons were never hers.

How much we castigate women for daring to *need*. How much I've learned, after everything, that the sin of caring too much about your daughters' problems is minor among the mistakes we humans make in love. How much more my own daughters have forgiven *me*, and yet here we are: still a family, I our matriarch now.

My sweat from the journey dries in the cool air. My daughters, nineteen and fit, joke how unexpectedly hard the hike up was, and I say a silent thank you to the mountain, the lake, my mother's ashes, that somehow I am here, at fifty-one, healthy, with a bionic hip that held.

Later, we walk on a glacier covered in flags from around the world, and something frozen inside me thaws further. Despite my divorce, my job loss, my cancer, my temporary disability and relentless pain, my feeling like some ancient temple in ruin amid my lightning-fast menopause that seemed at first to add insult to injury: I have been supporting my children for years now as a visiting lecturer with a recently launched consulting business; my memoir recently sold; I am about to reenter the PhD program I left twenty years prior. Life did not stop for any challenges, and at times this felt harrowing, unmanageable…but here, from a remove, I am able to see the beauty of that constant movement, too, shaping me the way water shapes stone.

* * *

The thing about my decade-long ride is that some variation of it comes for everyone. Someday, maybe I will get cancer again, and—cancer or not—someday I, too, will die. But when the ride comes for me again, I hope this time, I will recognize the carnival conductor as my kindred. I hope this time, we will greet each other as old friends, and instead of fighting and feigning, I will keep an open heart—even amidst pain—to what the ride is trying to show me.

Once upon a time, in early 2016, I conjured up a hyperbolically sexually dominant version of myself in order to survive the changes in my body—in my life. At first, this felt like vigilant performance art, much like the artificially strong and happy versions of myself that I once spoon-fed my mother. But over time, parts of that Me grew roots inside my psyche and stuck organically, integrated themselves into my fantasies, my multitudes, along with the reemergence of older desires, as well as entirely new terrain.

Whatever weak and pitiful thing I feared myself to be and overcompensated for in the bedroom, I was never that woman—any more than I was the easy daughter, the loyal first-and-forever wife. I am not static.

I am something else entirely that I am still uncovering.

FINDING MENO: LITTLE CLOWNS

By Monica Drake

Each morning, I reclaim my body, moving into a new day: I live here, in my particular biological system, in the solar system, in my mind and in my skin, traveling through time. Existence is laced with everyday miracles. I'm grateful to carry along the spirit and muscle memory of the girl I've always been, running wild through the woods, creeks, and fields, and later city streets, alleys, dark clubs. I've changed with age, moving into menopause, and I'm doing just fine. My hair, streaked with silver, is hippie child long, witchy long, crone long, left to be as it grows. I never have bothered much with haircuts.

I think more often about animals and insects, all kinds of love and the grace of existence. Lately, I've been considering clownfish. They're common and cute, swimming in oceans and saltwater tanks, hanging around reefs in a symbiotic relation-ship with sea anemones. One variation is brilliant orange with bold white stripes and black eyes as shiny as caviar. I'd love a dress with such strong graphics. We all know the look—it's Nemo, in *Finding Nemo*. The interesting thing is that clown-fish are born male, every last one. That creates disastrous sur-vival odds, with potentially no reproductive hope. They're still around because of their ability to change.

These fish remind us that change is natural. Change is a sur-vival skill.

Nemo would be born a sequential hermaphrodite. Given the right social cues, he might undergo a hormonal shift. His tiny fish testes would dissolve. His ovaries would grow. He'd carry and drop eggs, and become Mom. Pixar might choose to recast his fish-voice, and a handful of protesters would gather. Ha!

In my mid- to late forties, I went to my OB-GYN for an annual checkup. I saw the same doctor who delivered our daughter seven years earlier, as I do every year. She spread a cool, clear gel over my lower abdomen, then ran an ultrasound wand over my belly. Squinting, she said, "Your uterus is so thin, I can barely see it."

This was a new development.

I lay, half naked, on the white paper on her narrow exam table and propped myself up on my elbows to get a look. She pointed at her screen, tracing a thin line. My uterus was a ghost. Some women bleed more heavily in perimenopause. My peri-ods were still regular, only lighter.

I was impressed with my body's particular efficiency. The

news was surprising, but it wasn't an illness. It was the physical announcement of a new stage in my reproductive life.

It's easy to frame the loss of fertility as a harbinger, some kind of death-before-death, the faded flower, the fallen fruit. It's not death though, any more than a fried chicken dinner is a death by heart attack decades before the heart attack. Death and decay are not gendered. One way or another, death comes for us all— eventually. I was fine! I'd moved from a reproductive being to a post-reproductive being, while remaining fully human.

I cruised home through Portland's quiet back streets, one hand on the steering wheel, one elbow on my open window. I'd been child-free by choice until I turned thirty-nine. Then I chose to become a mother. As a mom I'm filled with daily love, gratitude, and amazement. I wouldn't want it any other way. I also will be okay continuing on this natural, biological arc.

I'd still be productive, just not reproductive.

As an undergrad, I studied animal behavior. As a kid, I grew up close to the earth. I've put my hands in the soil, collected water from swamps, seen praying mantises hatch by the hundreds, lived with an eye toward microscopic creatures and new-born elephants, too. I'm in love with the unfolding mystery of existence. By my late forties, I was still absolutely strong, compassionate, empathetic, and alive. I could shed a little conventional, youthful femininity. What did it matter?

Over the years of taking care of the house and family, I'd also written three books and designed and launched an undergraduate writing program for the college where I taught. Now, on my drive home from the gynecologist, after that delicate line of uterus showed itself, I medicated against any flicker of existential or mortal unease with a refreshed vision, a poultice of love, creativity, and opportunity: It was time to apply for a sabbatical, a break from teaching, to focus on my own creative work. I'd supported thousands of students. Now, I'd move toward a new dimension of purpose and personal freedom. In perimenopause, I resolved to claim a few more hours of my own, each day.

It took about two years before my sabbatical application was approved. In a span of the mildest of hot flashes, as I neared fifty, I gained permission for one year off from teaching and a half-year's pay. A modicum of freedom coupled with enough money to keep the bills paid would be the biggest life change of all. My husband earned a union hourly wage at the county library. Our family would be fine. I was humming along, taking care of everyone, doing all I could. My entire adult life I'd worked to get to this point.

But then on a summer's day, in the long fingers of an evening sun, on a day of heat and sprinklers, fountains in the park, in the months before my sabbatical officially began, as I looked forward to a fantastic future, writing and living, my husband came home in a rage. His mouth was a flat line. He poured a jelly jar full of wine and took a swig like it was water. His anger was free ranging, searching for a place to land. One way or another, I knew it would land on me, was already aimed at me, critical and scrutinizing.

Within the hour, he raged against a scholarship I'd secured to send our daughter to a local wilderness day camp. I wasn't sending her off to sleepaway camp, and definitely wasn't abandoning her. It was only a great, active, and relatively economical way for a ten-year-old to pass a few summer days outdoors, learning survival skills with other kids in a nearby wooded nature area.

He was walking fury, white-faced and rage-fueled. He followed me through the house, yelling, puffing up his chest, standing too closely. He had a list of accusations. The specifics of the list didn't matter, because each one was only an excuse for aggression. He put on a performance, attempting to exact subordination, my humiliation, in front of our child. He wanted our daughter to see her mother terrified. How do I know it was a performance for our daughter? Because between berating me, looming, and intimidating, he addressed her. He said, "Your mama! Your mama gets away with too much!"

Later he'd call this a "lesson."

In a panic, terrified at what was unfolding, I asked, "What do I get away with?"

That day, I'd taken our child to swim team practice. I'd made dinner. I was a workhorse—an author and a professor as well as a good mother, good wife, good friend. Not that even essential laziness would justify abuse. His fists were a threat. He'd been violent before. In the worst of times he once hit my head into a wall, held me by the throat. I thought we were past the nightmares. Most of the time, he could be a pretty cool guy?

He'd gone to counseling. I couldn't relate to or understand his irrational violence. He had so many reasons to be happy and grateful. All I knew was that once he let it fly, there was no way to quell his rage. He behaved as though compelled, like a rapist ejaculating. There's no other way to put it. I say rapist, because these episodes were not consensual or equal. They were imposed and unstoppable. His violent rage seemed to need a physical release. Afterward, it left me feeling emotionally battered and sometimes physically harmed.

This summer night in the time shortly before my sabbatical was to start, one of his rage storm ejaculations was coming on strong. "Your mama gets away with too much!"

I pleaded with him to take a breath, take a walk, wait it out and talk later, as adults, and most of all to leave our child out of it. But that's not the release he wanted. He wanted to be witnessed. He was enacting his violence in front of our child, because that was the kind of father he chose to be. He was trying to teach our daughter a gendered lesson of power, submission, and second-class citizenship, using my body as his rhetorical device. I didn't let it happen.

He kept up his diatribe, threats, and posturing. At some point I lifted my cell phone and began to film. I had no plan other than a sense that he should see himself, later, while in a calmer state of mind. He was having a fit. He needed help. We needed to escape. He was responsible for his own behavior. My concern was to stay safe and minimize drama, for our child's sake. I had to appear calm. I had to be smart and keep thinking and try to get us both safely out of the house. He lunged at me, while I stood on a set of cement stairs outside our back door. He grabbed my arm and knocked me off balance. I teetered on the stairs. There was no railing, only a pile of construction debris down below, broken glass, sharp scrap metal, and rusty nails on the cement walkway. I fought to get out of his grip but held on, too, to keep from falling. He pulled on the phone, prying my fingers, twisting my arm. I didn't let go. A phone is a lifeline to safety. I was working on surviving, one moment to the next. He was terrifying—and he wanted me to be terrified. I never understood the limits of his violence. There was no way to be sure he wouldn't kill me, either on purpose or by accident. I was trying to make my marriage work, but he wasn't a man anyone should be married to. When I couldn't get out of his grip, I shouted to the high heavens for help, as loudly as I could, hoping a neighbor would hear.

My husband let go and ran inside.

Soon after, he went to use the bathroom. I saw our chance. I had my keys, my phone. I whispered, "Run."

Our daughter and I hightailed it to the car in unison. He came after us. I locked the doors. He pounded on the windows. I put my foot on the gas. That was the end of our family constellation. I never went home to the house again, as long as he was there.

He sent texts accusing me of kidnapping. We stayed at the neighbors' house. I lay awake, in the night sweats of menopause, on a hot summer night, in the neighbor's back bedroom, watching their son's gecko cling to a branch where it lived in a tank under a blue light. My husband went to the hospital and reported that he'd been attacked. He showed them a small scratch, like something his own fingernail or one of the blackberry vines in our yard might bring about. They gave him a dollop of antibacterial ointment, smaller than a fast food ketchup packet, along with a note, *Do you feel safe at home?*

"You'll never see our daughter again!" he wrote, in an email. Thankfully, she was with me. He was unhinged. All I could assess with any degree of certainty is that he wasn't behaving as a physically or psychologically safe person to be around, ever again. He was willing to lie and eager to fight, treating me as though I were an enemy. The battle was his, not mine.

His anger didn't abate after most of a week. Our daughter and I stayed away, then after a week I asked him to leave the house so we could go home for a bit. He refused. He wasn't apologetic, was only waiting to finish what he'd started. Reluctantly, I filed for a restraining order. Police escorted him out. He hired a lawyer to contest the order. Specifically, he hired a "men's rights" lawyer, as though inflicting violence and ongoing aggression fell under the purview of men's rights. Once he'd lawyered up, as they say, I was compelled to hire a lawyer in response.

That's how I came to be waiting in the lobby of a law office, watching clownfish in a tank drifting up then darting down. They were so calming. Little clowns. I watched the little clowns.

If given the chance, those dreamy swimming glimmers of light and color would make their home in sea anemones, hanging out in the waving tendrils. Clownfish will shove smaller fish, minnows, right into the maw of an anemone, to feed their living home, their camouflage, their little duck blind as a hunter might say, protecting their corner of the ocean. Though they looked so mild as a species, they're opportunistic, both collaborative and predatory.

Heat rose from my chest into my neck and spread over my face. In that hot and harried week of summer, it seemed I'd moved into full-on menopause. I medicated a hot flash by rolling a cold can of sparkling water over my wrist. I didn't have time to think about my own body. This was a time for prioritizing others, namely our child. I had a lot to learn about the legal system.

My lawyer advised me to file for divorce. She said, "That way, the judge will know you're serious and be more likely to keep the restraining order in place."

I filed.

At first I thought it was a coincidence that I found myself with two distinct, equally significant life changes at once. One was violence, unkindness, and divorce—which weighed heavily on my heart and kept me looking over my shoulder. The second major concern was my own internal, hormonal terrain. Menopause had begun relatively easily. But with the fear and strain in our marriage, and then adding in lawyers, shifting hormones had started to tax my days, bringing a new level of exhaustion. Hot flashes were overwhelming, burning my chest from inside, coming on in waves then dissipating. I practiced breathing through them. They were also visible, and unstoppable. Each time a round of heat came on, the skin on my chest and my neck in particular would bloom bold red.

Here's what I didn't yet know—it turns out that the two concerns are deeply linked. The overlap wasn't coincidence. Domestic violence increases the "bothersome" effect of menopausal symptoms. It has to do with the endocrine system. As one study articulates, "Emotional intimate partner violence and posttraumatic stress [are] associated with sleep-related, vasomotor, and vaginal symptoms; physical intimate partner violence [is] associated with night sweats; and sexual assault [is] associated with vaginal symptoms."

We're engineered to live in community. Violence is a threat. Our bodies respond. Hot flashes, night sweats, insomnia, dry mouth, anxiety—it all grew increasingly difficult. Symptoms clawed at my insides as I stayed up night after night working through the litigious divorce.

What I also didn't know, as I moved into the stream of the courts, is that the court itself has an eighty-year history of faulting, blaming, shaming, and economically shortchanging women specifically for their menopausal experience. That's an alignment, intentionally or not, with a history of misogyny, age-ism, and financial abuse.

Unwittingly, I carried my menopausal body into the court-room, armed only with a sense that anyone would see an obvi-ous need for a mother to protect a child. I expected those paid to oversee divorce court to follow the basics of the legal sys-tem. I thought feminism held a little more traction, in valuing women as fully human, with economic and bodily autonomy rights, a right to safety and a right to an equitable division of assets earned throughout the marriage. It seems I was idealistic.

In a piece called "On Mirrors and Gavels: A Chronicle of How Menopause Was Used as a Legal Defense Against Women," by Phyllis T. Bookspan and Maxine Kline, the authors coin the term "the Menopause Defense" to refer to over fifty legal cases, ranging from about 1900 to the 1990s, in which women were financially devalued in court due to being anywhere at all on the continuum of having a relationship to menopause, from perimenopause to postmenopausal. It was specifically used in four kinds of cases, including personal injury and insurance cases, workman's compensation, tainted products, and divorce court. In these cases, menopause often reads as an accusation. It's shorthand, code for socially approved economic devaluation, conveniently lobbed at women anywhere from thirty-five to sixty—which is to say the prime earning years, roughly most anywhere in the span of an entire career.

In 1900, the medical industry knew even less about menopause than they do now. To bring the Menopause Defense into a court required no specifics—no medical exam or blood work, no concern with ascertaining that the woman was actually in menopause. It was only necessary to say that she probably was, and to bring on a whole slew of assumptions. The court relied on standard clichés about women and their bodies, specifically the commonly held, deeply misguided belief that menopause was a time when women went "crazy" and generally became unreliable, unstable, irritable, fragile, and prone to obscure health grievances, both physiological and psychological, well worth ignoring. In other words, most women could be discredited for being adult women past their twenties. The cases range from addressing events with very clear, physical bodily harm to interpersonal arguments, but most consistently aim toward discrediting, devaluing, and victim blaming. The article, along with corresponding court documents, offers a window into the mad-house of misogyny.

As one example, in 1900 a woman was run over by a horse pulling an ice wagon. Her bones were broken, including her ribs and neck, and her organs were damaged. The company that owned the horse blamed her problems on...menopause. Other women were subjected to gas leaks, poisoned foods, chemical burns, and more. Each case laid the foundation for the next corporation or disgruntled spouse to deflect blame, to point toward menopause as the source of all ailments.

Before no-fault divorce became law, menopause was used as an excuse to justify abandonment, affairs, neglect, and some-times violence. As the authors of the study point out, the highest use of the Menopause Defense in the court system in the United States was during World War II, as women entered the job force and men joined the military. Women were gaining economic ground; their essential biology was used to disenfranchise them from economic settlements more frequently than in any other time. "The menopause defense...was an overt, bold and accepted means to devalue women's injuries, damages, and life worth."

The Menopause Defense relies on a tacit cultural and legal agreement of devaluation: Women's bodies and lives are viewed as inherently worthless.

The most recent cited use of the Menopause Defense, in the article, was in 1995. The Cracker Barrel restaurant tried to dodge liability for a "slip and fall" by claiming the injury sustained was "common in postmenopausal women."

The judge who oversaw our divorce graduated from law school in 1996, one year after that last Menopause Defense effort. She was a woman who survived an education in a system of male privilege and gendered body shame, age shame, femininity shame. She found her way up the ladder under the ordinary constraints of patriarchy. From what I saw, as I came to know her through years in her courtroom, she'd learned how to play the game.

Court is haunted with a history and framework of misogyny. Too many gendered clichés are still treated as though true. There are laws in place, designed to encourage a culture of equity, parity. Laws have wiggle room, though. Ultimately they're only as good as the people sworn to uphold them.

In court, I was identified in all caps, as WIFE and MOTHER. That was my identity and my role.

There were three separate paths of court dates. My ex contested the initial restraining order, twice. That process took it from the county court to the state supreme court, and lasted longer than the order itself, which is to say over a year. It was easily upheld, clearly necessary and legitimate. The second thread of court dates involved renewing the restraining order, after the first year, when the first one expired. The renewal was considered a second order. My ex contested it again. The renewed restraining order process overlapped with the year or so it took for the first restraining order to get to the state supreme court, creating two different judicial paths and sets of dates to track. Then there was divorce court, which was separate from either restraining order case.

The need for first one lawyer, then eventually another, came on as unexpectedly as menstrual spotting, in ways that were very real, yet also as surreal as the suffocating, internal, ghostly hand I often felt as though at my throat, strangling me from the inside, in a hot flash.

Court dates came on like cluster headaches, overriding my ability to consider my own work, interrupting parenting and time with family. If I missed a court date for a restraining order, an Order of Protection, the order would be dropped, and my ex could come back to the house. Notification for these court dates didn't always reach me, though. At times the announcement of an upcoming date in court was sent to the wrong email, the wrong lawyer, the wrong place. It was a steady threat. At least once, I missed a court date I'd never known was scheduled. Then I petitioned, asked for forgiveness, asked for another round, jumped back in...Rooms for the hearings were scheduled then rescheduled, sometimes in different buildings miles apart.

I made a doctor's appointment, for my own health, and canceled it. Who has the time?

Instead, I rushed one way, then the other, to court. Most often we met at the courthouse downtown. Other times, for the convenience of the judge, we were scheduled where she also worked, in the Juvenile Justice center. It was often unclear and shifting, where and when court proceedings would occur. My job was to drop everything, sometimes turning the car around on my way to work, and to show up looking ready for business, ready to tolerate claims against my being, ready to be patient and to pay out by the thousands in legal fees for my own bodily and economic protection and in the ongoing effort toward divorce.

I entered into the court system, single parenting and swamped in visible hot flashes, awash in the kind of sleeplessness that comes from busy days and long nights spent sorting out divorce documents, visibly menopausal, visibly exhausted. I would say that I came to court with what some might call "resting bitch face," but I was not resting. I was listening, watching, squinting, learning, pausing, trying, parenting, fleeing, living, sweating, shedding, hoping, worried about paying legal fees, surviving, in menopause, in life. I was not resting. I definitely wasn't smiling.

Should I have smiled?

I swore to tell the truth while the pale skin of my chest and neck blazed with the combustion of a human animal shapeshifting. I laid a hand against the cool, blonde wood and left a handprint, sweating like a criminal.

Lawyers advise clients to dress conservatively, take off unconventional piercings, hide tattoos. A woman's furrowed forehead can read as too angry. A loud voice, a raspy voice, a significant breast enlargement, a highly feminized presence, a pink handbag, a tendency to blink or flinch or look away, these all potentially feed into conclusions drawn by a judge. I'd consider these superficial social signifiers, but in court every cough and stutter is scrutinized. The judges consider presentation as part of context and content.

I couldn't hide that flush of heat, the chemistry of the body and its wealth of emotions. I let the rising wave wash through me, reminding myself that the suffocating sensation was transitory. It would disperse.

There are two parts to divorce in a marriage with children: child custody arrangements and the division of assets. My husband gave up custody. He chose not to go in front of the judge. I became the sole legal parent, there to make all medical and educational decisions, among other aspects. He gave that up?

My lawyer said, "He doesn't want the judge to see that video..."

We live in a no-fault state, like most states in the United States. This meant that his threatening behavior wouldn't be considered or discussed, in terms of dividing our finances. To mention his violence would be viewed as trying to "fault" him, which was off the table. It would only be justifiable to present his actions if we were discussing his parenting. A smart judge, my lawyer said, would notice that he gave up custody so readily and read between the lines.

The first part of the division of assets process is called Discovery. This involves turning over documentation of all accounts. I handed over my docs in a quick afternoon. Boom! Done.

What we "discovered" in Discovery was that my estranged husband essentially followed an aggressor's playbook of violence. He hid money, moved money, shuffled through bank accounts, piled up debt, lied when it was convenient. He went after my father's house, costing me thousands of dollars and mental anguish. He made a list of things he imagined he was owed, including an approximately three-dollar, very old, very ordinary box cutter. He returned to his list repeatedly, at the cost of a combined five to six hundred dollars an hour in legal fees, more than enough to buy plenty of box cutters. He hid his retirement account's value, then formally requested to take mine, which was much smaller. He wanted all of everything. His rage was irrational, his relationship to finances was terrible.

He turned off the utilities in our house, where our daughter and I lived. I'd paid the bills. He took the time to make phone calls, to have everything shut off, leaving us suddenly without electricity, heat, or internet access. He pocketed the refunds and deposits, which I'd paid. I spent more money to have every-thing turned back on. Apparently this is a move used so fre-quently that it's diagnostic. It's a bullet point on a pamphlet put together by the county, illustrating how to identify abusive tac-tics: shutting off utilities.

He totaled his car in a one-person accident, in a way that I'd say reeked of booze, to the soundtrack of glass breaking, bottles rattling. I wasn't there, but I knew him well. In court, he tried to capitalize on the accident by using it to move his car off the chart of assets. He said it was no longer an asset. My lawyer tracked down the mechanic where it was being repaired—because it was still of value. She called him out in court. My ex's behavior turned everything into an expensive game of Unveil the Lies.

Somewhere in the battering headwind of ongoing court dates, there evolved a riff that I was considered "bad with money." My hard-won sabbatical was treated as an economic indul-gence, reducing my salary, rather than a fleeting honor actively obliterated as court rolled forward, taking up all time and emotional, psychological landscape.

Weaponizing the court system, prolonging proceedings, causing additional stress and expense, is a standard abuser's tactic.

In truth, I'm a former mortgage underwriter for two major banks. Underwriting was a well-paying job I bounced into after grad school. I'd started as a temporary receptionist and moved quickly to making major lending decisions because the people at the top saw that I'm good with details and guidelines. I have a strong understanding of reasonable versus unreasonable calculations of income, debt, and risk. My credit scores are high.

I'd earned $100,000 on a book deal in the years before my sabbatical. I earned $58,000 a year at the college where I was full time. Reducing my teaching load was a calculated gamble based on having earned more through writing than I would in one year of teaching, and as an added benefit, I'd work toward being the writer I set out to be so many years before.

With or without saying the words, in the cultural imagination women fill the role of "spenders" and "gold diggers." I was advised not to "go after" my husband's money, when I pointed out his basic inconsistencies. In court, I was able to demonstrate his financial misrepresentations more than once. As an underwriter, it had been my job to make sure all of a lender's docs were in. I found a statement showing most of $1 million—$891,000 dated back a few years earlier—which had mysteriously not been mentioned. Every underwriter knows the importance of a paper trail. Under oath, my estranged husband told the court that money just didn't exist. Nobody asked him to produce the paper trail. Poof! Like magic, the document and all the questions it raised effectively disappeared from discussion. The court treated his answers as legitimate and reasonable. If I asked about it again, my lawyer let me know I'd be seen as an angry wife, placing unreasonable demands on my ex.

On a break, I soaked a rough, courthouse paper towel in cold water and pressed it to my forehead. I was awash in menopausal hormones, in a sea of gendered mechanics based on financial entitlement and power, which is to say very specifically the stories that build the essential armature of patriarchal capitalism.

His "men's rights" lawyer took the kind of risks my lawyer did not, willing to try to fault me, under a no-fault process. Though we couldn't discuss violence, I was challenged, questioned, for some vague, unsubstantiated assertion that I had a propensity toward buying the family organic lettuce.

While my body navigated the terrain of menopause, court became the place where my husband was allowed to denigrate me in public, the ground always shifting and surging.

The court exists in a symbiotic relationship with the aggrieved. My ex had a bruised ego. I was the minnow, shoved in the anemone's maw, to feed the paychecks and pay the bills of lawyers and the judge, keeping everything moving as it has for centuries.

All I wanted was out.

That dry mouth feeling of panic under pressure? It's the same, essentially, as the dry mouth of menopause. It's what a dental hygienist referred to as xerostomia. While people are writing editorials about vaginal dryness—valuing and highlighting a vagina for its receptivity to penetrative sex—a woman's mouth, at midlife, is shifting in ways worth discussion, and in need of increased care.

In court, my husband's financial micromanaging and stalking was portrayed as financial wisdom. I couldn't make my own financial choices through the years of the divorce court process.

Off the witness stand, from a stiff chair in the courtroom, I ran a tongue over my teeth, sipped water and listened. My estranged husband used a calm voice. His lawyer asked him to quantify the economic value of a decade of my childcare— considering it separately from, say, my household income, which had grown larger than his, and separately from thousands of meals, the labor of housework, the inherent value of love and friendship, while ignoring any essential moral and legal concerns of considering one person's lifetime as another person's economic asset. They discussed my life as though I'd been unpaid household help.

My then-husband said, "I never thought of it as a financial benefit to me, to have Monica at home. I mean, it was what she wanted to do..."

I had an unpaid internship in housekeeping hell, in his little paradigm. He generously let me take care of everything.

Childcare is a $60 billion industry, in the United States. I helped our family avoid spending, as much as we could, to make it easier for everyone and to save the money that was now considered his.

My ex and his lawyer reduced my body to a job site. I was an asset that had failed to hold value, a failed investment. I gulped from the glass of water then refilled it from a pitcher and drank again, dousing body heat and grief.

The soft skin of my lower belly was marked with the raised smile of a scar, an emergency C-section, a four-minute, ragged, and potentially life-threatening surgery. Court was a theater of misogyny. My reproductive years had come to a close. My life, though, had most definitely not.

We were working from two wildly different belief systems, two different stories. I saw midlife and beyond as a chance to shine. He saw it as a time to turn me into a diminished, battered, and subordinated narcissist's discard. I'd worked for decades and finally crafted a life with a bit of time and money; my ex set out to ensure I'd have neither. He didn't like the idea that I would have a sabbatical, a break from labor.

It cost us both hundreds of thousands of dollars to assuage his rage.

The judge most certainly had the means to read between the lines.

In the end, she awarded him all of our joint finances, overlooked the mysterious most-of-$1 million, which he said didn't exist, and required me to pay him for half of our home without offsetting that cost by the hundreds of thousands of joint finances he was holding onto. The judge made domestic violence vastly lucrative.

My lawyer asked, "Wouldn't those funds offset—"

The judge said, "She doesn't get any [money]. She's a spender, she spent hers." It was as though the judge herself was a financial abuser, doling out an allowance instead of trusting my informed, adult, and reasonable economic choices.

I picked at the sleeve of my nine-dollar Sears unlined suit. That suit was a bargain of a prop. I'd worn it too many days in a row. I'm a Goodwill shopper and a mostly DIY renovator, a writer, a homebody, a cook, and frugal. The judge saw a woman and assumed a poor relationship to finances. She made a wealthy man out of a violent man.

If I were a creature with a biological ability to naturally change gender—and there are many out there—court would've been a good time to make that change for purely practical reasons, economic reasons, culturally conditioned gender role reasons, to turn off the flickering film that played over my body, over all women's bodies, in the collective imagination of highly gendered projection and devaluation.

Money is never only money. In the court system, and against a background of restraining orders, money very clearly represents the ability to hire a lawyer, to stay safe.

To strip me of all finances was to bind me to the roles of WIFE and MOTHER, which could also be said as TARGET and LESS and SUBHUMAN, through the lens of my ex's aggression. When the judge offered her far-flung, nonconforming decision, my lawyer bit her lip. She laid a hand on my arm. She hiss-whispered, "This is not how the law works—"

Ten days later, my lawyer returned to court with a four-page brief. She requested the judge reopen the case and consider recusing herself.

We were granted a hearing.

On the day of that extra hearing, my ex wasn't there. His law-yer was a scratchy voice over the speakerphone. Neither could make time to come in.

The judge asked that I leave the courtroom. She wanted to consult with the lawyers privately. I listened to their voices through the courtroom door. My sabbatical had long since been obliterated. I had classes to teach, a life to manage. The judge asked that the basic tenets of divorce law be articulated for her.

My lawyer explained divorce law fundamentals. The judge fell apart. "You're right, I'm sorry!" she said. "I'm sorry! I did not do my job right." The lack of a contraction in those words? It's how she spoke, as though to enunciate each syllable of her fail-ing. It's how her words read in the court transcript now.

The judge said, "I thought we had this sort of...tacit agreement."

A tacit agreement is an *unspoken* agreement. The reason it is unspoken is because it's the terrain of personal or cultural prej-udice, not law.

What was the tacit agreement she believed existed?

The ghost of the menopause defense moved past in a cool breeze. It oozed from the heavy bench in the hallway, the old building, the voices through the door, the scratch of the men's rights lawyer squawking over the speaker. I could be wrong. At times, one can only guess. That's the thing about ghosts— you can't quite see them, but you can sure sense something is there, usually something old, creepy, and presumably long passed...

The judge's decision was not remotely in accordance with

the legal practice of divorce. She knew better and caved quickly, but it didn't change the economic outcome.

It seemed she believed there was a common understanding that a woman was fair game for devaluation and a man was entitled to more than his share of the family finances.

Though nobody said the word "menopause," I'm going to say that this judge, an older woman, may have seen in me only her own learned self-loathing.

People who carry unbearable shame create scapegoats to serve as a vessel, a place to put their least manageable emotions. I believe that in her courtroom I was a stand-in for women in general, surviving at the nexus of misogyny, ageism, and hot flashes. The judge used her authority to try to craft a scapegoat, perhaps to imagine that her life in a woman's body was different, better, less failable than all the others.

Your mama gets away with too much...

You're right, I'm sorry...I did not do my job right...I thought we had a tacit agreement...

It didn't change anything, financially. It didn't rewind time or put money in the bank. But it's rare to receive an apology from a judge. My lawyer was astounded.

Bring up menopause now that I'm on the other side of all that, and my mind races with residual trauma. I'm working to let the flashbacks go. "Oh, my god—all the lawyers, right? What...a...*nightmare*."

When people talk about the symptoms of menopause, the conversation leans toward the biological and psychological, how we feel and manage. Beyond these parameters though, beyond the individual, there's an entire additional assembly of sociocultural menopausal symptoms. From the OB-GYN's office, I definitely hadn't foreseen the larger institutional, cultural control aspects coming on.

There are generations of women who learned to view menopause as something to hide, and something to loathe. Too many are still carrying that learned shame, unfortunately willing to pass it on to the next generation.

There's body shame locked in old stories, on a history of heavy rotation. Those are the stories of an oppressive system, of body-othering, body shaming, diminishing, and dismissing. Menopause shame, like period shame and weight shame, is a toxic river running through degraded generations, and it carries into the economic and other aspects of lives of women, children, the courts, the law.

I'd like to experience menopause without patriarchal capitalism breathing its hot breath of entitlement and rage. As it is, I cannot separate the bodily memory of rising and falling internal heat, like a suffocating hand, from the external hand of my husband as he reached for my wrist, twisting my arm on a summer night, trying to wrestle away the phone that I needed to call for help.

We live in systems, not isolation. The limbic system is a set of brain structures that involve our emotions, including the emotions of parenting, maternal bonding, and memories, but also love and sex. The limbic system works in concert with the emotional landscape of those around us, with a laugh or a look, a scent. The limbic system is also what scientists call "rich in estrogen receptors." An interpersonal assault and a hostile environment coupled with diminishing estrogen levels may potentially create a very specific effect on the forebrain, heightening menopausal symptoms in concert with community.

With clownfish, the hormonal changes that trigger a gender transition come on through social shifts. The exact genetic mechanism of microbiology that speaks from one fish-body to the others is still mystifying. That's the magic. Researchers are working on it. How does the death of a female signal to the hormonal chemistry of the largest male of the group? What is being conveyed between genes, in genetic messaging, from one to another? It involves both the brain and gonads, they say. And why don't others in the school of fish change, too? Somehow, collectively, their bodies know whose job it is. Their bodies are in sync. The others move one spot up in a hierarchy, though subordinate to the new Mom and Dad. They wash the eggs in their own mouth, then protect their clutch, little clown sentries.

Clownfish are far from utopian, though. Only one male mates with the sole female. If you have as few as three clownfish in a tank, they'll become a bullying triad, bullying the third into subordination. It takes a school of underlings to be safe, or none at all.

In court I lost my life savings. I lost years. Everyone else in the courtroom earned a significant income by bullying me into subordination and economic exploitation. Every lawyer, the judge, my ex. I was the sole financial minnow. I was the only woman in court in a menopausal body, and I was actively devalued. Money means power, in that bullshit system.

But in life, stories also hold power.

I'm grateful to know that I operated with integrity, and aimed only to make good choices, not to exploit or undermine anyone else. My story is clean.

From where I am now, I can look back and see a lineage of women in court overtly faulted for living in women's bodies, particularly in menopause. I can see my own days as they unfolded, and I can see the women coming after me, after us, into the future. The biggest change—THE CHANGE—right now is in telling the stories, real stories. True stories about lived lives forge cultural change.

There's deep work to be done, and lighthearted living.

When we say THE CHANGE, the biggest change is the one that is taking place right now, in releasing body shame, reproductive health shame.

As for me, I've survived. I'm strong, healthy, happy to be myself rather than anyone else in that courtroom, and best of all, I'm so vibrantly alive.

THE WOMAN AT THE REGISTER

By Lan Samantha Chang

Appleton, Wisconsin, 1991. It's a bright, cool northern summer afternoon. I'm reading in the passenger seat of our family station wagon while my father runs an errand at the hardware store. Or is it the bakery? No matter, because they're the same: potential settings of turbulence and drama.

I'm twenty-six years old, visiting my parents, and I'm reading *A Room of One's Own*. I've vowed to be a writer; and I'm in the process of carving out the parts of my life that do not fit this vow.

The power locks shoot open. My father gets into the car and slams the door. He is a mercurial man—a tempestuous, vehement man. Even his silence thunders, fumes.

What is it? What has upset him? I stare out the window,

focus on tracing the bright-edged clumps of the box elder leaves against the sky.

"*That woman!*" he shouts, in his sonorous baritone.

"What woman? At the counter?"

"At the *register*. The *clerk*."

A native speaker of Mandarin, an immigrant of four decades, my father prides himself on knowing the specific English words for titles, ranks, positions. Equally quick is his tendency to take offense whenever social rules are broken. I close my book, steel myself against his impending detonation. Part of my desire to be a writer lies in the appeal of coolness, distance. A solitary room, a life in which these interactions are not mine. But my curiosity overrides this desire.

I venture, "What about her?"

"When women reach *that age!*" The air between us rings. "When women reach that age, they just give up! They don't even care about pleasing people anymore!"

Years later, when I related this story, my oldest sister said our father's rage was not directed toward postmenopausal women per se. "It's aesthetic," she said. "He loved beauty. He was offended when any woman didn't care about making herself look good."

This could be true. My father's aesthetic ideals were inspired by his decades-long submersion-by-screen into the gender-binary principles of early television, old films, documentaries about political heroes and their wives. He consumed voraciously this mid-century culture, found aesthetic pleasure in its images. When they were dating, he took dozens of photos of my lovely young mother dressed in sweaters and pencil skirts, poised lightly against fountains, walls, automobiles. And he liked blondes, especially Grace Kelly with her slender elegance and shining hair. He admired Deborah Kerr enough to give his oldest daughter the middle name of Deborah.

Perhaps the woman's behavior was simply a racist micro-aggression. But my sister and I suspected it was not; at least, it wasn't the confrontational kind of male racism I'd seen my father handle with surprising grace. This happened when I was about ten years old. We were leaving the Kohl's, my father walking ahead of me clutching a bag, traveling in that liminal space between the first and second set of doors. I was behind him. The customer ahead of him, a taller, hefty man, went through the outer door, then turned and shoved it closed, physically shut the plate glass door against my father. Then opened it; we stumbled out. The man looked at my father straight in the face and said, "I've seen enough like you in Korea!"

Nothing more; they went their separate ways.

"What was that about?" I asked him, angry on his behalf. "What is he talking about? You're not Korean; you're Chinese."

My father glowered—not at the stranger, but at me. "You don't know anything," he said. And in his voice, and in the way he strode to the car, I could tell that he was deeply, darkly angry; but I also felt somehow he was protecting this stranger against my ignorance of history, that he understood this man and, perhaps, had encountered men like him before.

My father accepted male aggression, but the indifference of the woman behind the register filled him with rage. His response to the hostile gesture of an unknown white man was nothing compared to his indignity, his frustration over an interaction with an older woman who didn't bother to fix herself up. To him, her short, naturally gray hair, evidence of a decision not to perm or color, was a sign that she didn't care what he thought. Her practical shoes represented a choice to pursue ugliness. These decisions were a rejection of aesthetic gratification, to him, a rejection of life. They transcended racism or cultural stereotypes. Her refusal to be pleasant with him was a human affront to him, it was personal.

A physically vigorous, handsome man in his late sixties at the time, a man of wit, with a classical Chinese education and an unconcealed emotional intensity, my father never had trouble getting attention from women. He dressed with simple elegance. He could be charming, he could follow the rules, and he wanted others to do the same.

In *A Room of One's Own*, Virginia Woolf wrote, "Women have served all these centuries as looking glasses possessing the magic and delicious power of reflecting the figure of man at twice its natural size." For my father, this woman's power worked in reverse. He couldn't bear her indifference. For she *was* indifferent. She had no interest in pleasing, not in the particular way that mattered to my father; perhaps she'd never had. Or perhaps she felt her days of being able to gain his sexual interest were past, so why should she bother?

He wanted attention. Maybe he joked with her about having perfect change and she didn't laugh at his joke. Or she hated waiting for customers to count out perfect change. Maybe he had a question, or a grievance couched as a question—*why* are they so often out of 75-watt bulbs?—and something in her answer struck him as lacking in care. Maybe she condescended to him—speaking too slowly, assuming, from his Asian features, that he was fresh off the boat. This would frustrate him. He'd try again—something a little more conspicuous this time, assuming she'd see he'd been in the United States for years. She was brusque with him, I have no doubt. And so he detonated. He raised his voice in a retort and stormed out, bringing dark clouds of anger and vexation to the car.

"She didn't even try!" he fumed, saying these words in English, in order to communicate to me as clearly as possible that the woman's lack of effort was contemptible. He was telling me not to become that woman, a woman who had reached an age at which the appearance of caring about traditional relationships with men was not a part of her life and who wasn't fighting it.

For years after the incident at the hardware store, I longed to be this unknown woman at the register. I wanted her short, gray hair. I craved a body that did not periodically steam and stink of my own fertility. I especially craved the indifference with which I would inhabit such a body. I worked to enact indifference. My great grandmothers in China bound their feet; I refused to wear uncomfortable shoes. I kept my hair short, my toenails natural, and my fingernails blunt.

My mother, whose story deserves to be told more fully, another time, nagged me so much about finding a boyfriend that I threatened to break off our relationship if she ever brought up the subject again. She didn't bring up the subject again. It is my father who pushed me, again in Wisconsin, winter now. We were in the frigid garage, digging out the snow shovels. I was in my thirties with no boyfriend. He turned to face me, yelled, "You're afraid of life!" And maybe he was right. I knew exactly what he meant by "life." It meant making the choices he'd made. It meant joining my life to others; it meant responsibility, it meant compromise.

For years, I didn't date anyone. I strove to reach a degree of solitude that would allow me to focus on my writing more than anything. No preoccupation, no passions. Only in this way could I concentrate. Only in this way would I reach what Woolf might call my truth. I tried to overlook the monthly burden of my financial precarity. To think of only reading and writing so that I wasn't tempted to stray into the equally vexing worry that I was wasting my life—that I'd almost literally put my eggs into one basket.

Woolf wrote of the peace achieved with her inheritance: "I need not hate any man; he cannot hurt me. I need not flatter any man; he has nothing to give me. So imperceptibly I find myself adopting a new attitude towards the other half of the human race." It is through finding this peace that I might touch the "freedom and full expression" that were the "essence of the art." But I had no inheritance; instead, my student loan payments surpassed my rent. I was not at peace. For this reason, I could not adapt any such peace toward others. I was ensnarled in not-so-secret longings, loneliness, anxiety. Nonsexual attachments, unexpected crushes and disappointments, complex, confusing friendships.

My attitude toward men was snarly, angry. I picked fights with people and refused to listen to my oldest sister, the middle name of Deborah: "Just flirt with them for five minutes," she said. "If you just flirt for five minutes, when you meet them, then they like you and you can get down to business. You can have a good working relationship." I detested her pragmatism.

I went for a walk with Anne, a coworker twice my age, in the hills behind Palo Alto. Anne lived alone in a small, pleasant, and pricey bungalow she'd purchased with the money left over from her marriage. She had two adult children, both out of college and living on their own. She had a job at the university where I was teaching—not a stressful job, but a place to go every day, people to talk to. As we climbed into the foothills, gaining perspective on the sun-drenched vista of yellow hills scattered with the dark green live oaks, she told me about her house and children. She talked about her twenty-three-year marriage, which had ended over ten years ago when her husband had fallen in love with another man and left her without ever telling her why; she'd gleaned the truth only from gossip. The knowledge upset her at first, she said, staring at the lion-colored hills. For a while, she found the truth of her marriage hard to accept. But now she could see that he refused to tell her not because of anything she had or hadn't done, as his wife, but because he was ashamed of how much he had lied to her. I gazed out at the foothills, admiring her age, experience, perspective. I craved her distance and content. Dreaded responsibilities—employment, partner, children— loomed, before I might be able to see behind me and before me with such clarity.

I yearned to skip over the middle of life entirely.

I was an adjunct instructor, still determined to be a writer, but yet to publish more than a couple of short stories. I had yet to fall in love. In contrast, Anne's life, post-love, seemed clean and spacious, even capacious. Her children were grown and her marriage ended. She had earned the right to say she'd partnered, she had mothered. The pressure to do these things was over and done with. This absence of pressure felt to me like absolute freedom. Yet I was, at that time, a woman of childbearing age, meaning that whenever I did not decide against children, did not take active measures to prevent children from happening, my life was capable, at any moment, of being hijacked by my own fertility. If I got pregnant, I would be faced with the decision about what to do. If I decided to have children, my life would be bound by that decision for twenty years.

I envied Anne her fewer choices. I told myself that I was made not for the turmoil of adulthood but for a peaceful old age.

And yet I was filled with anxiety about my future. I dreaded responsibility, suspecting I was destined to have it. And might want it. Although I didn't wish to change myself, didn't wish to compromise, I longed for someone who wanted to throw in their lot with me. Anne and I discussed my emotional problems. She thought that if I only found a partner, my life would click satisfactorily into a stable pattern of marriage, family-building. I did want this, but I wanted more: some path into the middle years in which I retained enough control over my own life to keep from losing my fragile writing practice. I needed more than a room of my own, as it turned out: I wanted to earn that room myself. I wanted to make enough money so I wouldn't ever be forced to please anyone.

Around this time, I jettisoned the idea of marriage as a source of any financial support.

Anne discussed her two children, very different, both independent; I envied her these grown children. They were hers, her accomplishments. Her time of active parenting was past and she talked about them as if they were entirely separate from her, but they were still tethered; they would always be *her children*. I knew this tether was hard-won. She had given up years of her life for them; she'd given up whatever youthful ambitions she had toward being a visual artist so that she could be there for them. I was told my generation was different from hers. I was told I could choose to have both children and writing. But deep down, I sensed it will be a mortal struggle, and I dreaded that struggle, with its accompanying sacrifice, which lay in the future.

I had to face the truth: that I envied Anne meant I didn't want to be Virginia Woolf. To want to have done it meant that I must do it. I must embark upon the middle of life with its illusions of partnership, family, responsibility, what I considered permanence.

One day, when we were walking, I told Anne: I sensed it was time to move forward and to live out my life, whatever it might be. But I also desired to delete the next thirty years. I wanted to outgrow the stage of needing or wanting to please men, ever. I wanted it all to be completed and in the past so I could focus on doing what I want to do.

Anne politely listened to my description of her life, and then she let out a cackling laugh.

She *was* proud of her children, her accomplishments, her home. The only problem, she told me, is that she still *did* care what men think of her. Our walks in the foothills were an essential part of her conditioning routine. She counted her steps and calories. Since menopause, her hair had thinned. Her short, lightly curled hairstyle, while appearing effortless, actually cost her a great deal of time and money. Every six weeks, she spent hours at the hairdresser coloring, clipping, curling. She spent more money on her hair than on any other part of her budget. So she was free, she said, but not entirely free.

In the end, I waited until almost the last possible moment to compromise. I waited until I'd published not one, but two books before I married at thirty-nine. I had my child, with help from doctors, when I was forty-two. My daughter is now sixteen, the joy of my life, and in a few weeks, I turn fifty-nine: the age of Virginia Woolf when she loaded her coat pockets with stones and walked into the River Ouse.

There's no perfect moment for change. My last menstrual period ended in 2014, the year of my mother's death. As a widower, my father embarked upon what one of my sisters would call a kind of solitary old bachelorhood in which he ate Kentucky Fried Chicken whenever he wanted, watched his favorite movies until all hours, and struggled alone in our family house like a zoo creature that has outlived its companions. I sometimes wish I could say that he and I gave each other solace and comfort in that time, but we did not. I spent a year too hurt to receive comfort from any older person. To deepen the sense of loss, two mentors at my university retired and one was losing his memory. The whole world was turning over and my body's transition seemed a bit like a natural response, a true stopping of all the clocks. That is how it felt to me: Losing menstruation felt, and still does feel, as if a steady rhythm, a beat of time, has been smoothed away from the texture of my life, and I am plunged so deeply into the chaos of everything I once dreaded that the years circle ever faster.

I did discuss losing my period at MacDowell, with a fellow writer, Molly. She said she missed the way her face used to look. She informed me, bluntly, that in five years, I would appear completely different. This did happen when I was too busy to notice. I can see it now, and I regret it, especially when I'm searching through my closet. I've gone gray. The colors of my skin and hair no longer make a clear contrast, so I can't wear the most vibrant shades I used to love.

The most unexpected change to happen with menopause is that I feel so much more at ease with men of all ages than I felt as a young woman. There are no stakes for me any more. I'm not as quiet or constrained with strangers; I often sense affection and a kind of love flowing out of me, and I can feel them accepting it and giving it back, quietly or happily, in return.

My father was afraid of death. I'd known this, sensed it somehow, since I was a small child. Perhaps it was this fear that caused him to need and want women to please him. For as long as the woman at the register looked, and acted, like a woman younger than she was, he would be a younger man. I can sympathize with that.

Toward the late middle age, he developed a heart condition. Periodically, he landed in the hospital and the nurses swarmed around him, teasing him at each shift and singing his praises whenever we visited. "Your father is a doll!" The first time this happened, I was utterly baffled. How could they believe this of him? And why wasn't he angry or impatient with the nurses, why did he submit himself so patiently and cheerfully to the innumerable indignities of being in the hospital? Not all of the nurses were pretty or young. But the dynamic was set: Their professional cheerfulness, their willingness to tease, put him into a good mood, despite his weakness, his vulnerability. After my mother was gone, the nurses kept him periodic company until his death at ninety-seven.

My sisters and I keep his bloodline flowing. We are all intense, forceful, witty, verbally expressive. None of us gave up work for family. We all practiced professions and were able to support ourselves. We gave birth to a total of six grandchildren. Eventually, we all reached the age of the woman at the register.

I have now spent close to twenty years working a full-time job, partnering, and mothering. I have written two novels in that time. I know my productivity is nothing close to what it might have been had I not chosen to compromise.

Still, I feel content. I wonder if I had so little trouble with menopause—some hot flashes, some weight gain, but no depression or insomnia, no feeling unlike myself—because my late arrival into the middle of life created a false sense of youth. Even now, I am still raising my child, surrounded by younger mothers, absorbed in activities that make me feel less than my age. I also reached menopause with a strong sense of relief and gratitude: relief that the pressures of my fertile years were clearly over; gratitude for my general health, for the luck of eventually finding a suitable mate, for the medical science that enabled me to have a child. Grateful that despite a long, troubled time, the procrastination, misery, and indecision that lasted through my youth, I was able to make it through middle age.

Sometimes, I know I have spent my life waiting for these years. Sometimes it is like being up in the hills, glimpsing the view.

Reimagining, Reinventing, Restorying

THE AFTERLIFE OF MENOPAUSE

By Julia Alvarez

On the day I turned fifty, I found myself in my walk-in closet, looking through my clothes. I'm a bit of a pack rat, saving what might prove useful down the road, if not for daily wear, then at the very least, for a dress-up theme party or a granddaughter's costume for Halloween. There were peasant blouses and long flowing hippy flower-child skirts; ethnic shawls and huipils; no-nonsense teaching attire to boost my credibility in the classroom: blazers and blouses, wool pants and skirts; several trophy-wife minimalist dresses with low necklines and short skirts that my husband liked to give me in tissue-layered boxes as gifts that he wanted to see me wear; even an ex-husband's sweatpants and sweatshirt I borrowed from his stash to try out his cure-all remedy for the funk I was in while married to him. "Nothing a good run won't lick." Running up and down the hills near our Oakland apartment never worked, but the depression did lift when I ran away from the good wife I mistakenly thought I could be.

You get the picture. That closet held the outfits that had dressed the different Julias I'd been, and which now lay nestled inside me like those Russian dolls. I ran my hand over these outfits wistfully and began culling the ones I no longer wanted to keep.

I don't think I'm alone in having been—and continuing to be, I might add—a multitude of selves. It just took me a long time—half a century—to embrace them all and not feel there was a "right one" to be. The female messaging had always been so restrictive and proscriptive. Growing up in the Dominican Republic in the 1950s in a strict Catholic family, we girls were taught that a woman's singular role was to be a wife and mother, or the allowable exception, if single, a nun or a lay version of nuns, an old-maid jamona who cared for her elders and extended familia. When we immigrated to the United States in the early sixties, my sisters and I went wild with the possibilities—quite circumscribed if judged by opportunities available now but given where we had come from, the opportunities seemed boundless. Of course, we had no idea how to handle all this freedom, but one thing was for sure, Mami and our Old World tías could no longer be our guides.

Being immigrants was actually similar to being female in a man's world: Both involved navigating a foreign culture where the dominant others wielded the power. Along with English, my sisters and I learned new ways to be and behave in order to belong and ultimately succeed. We ended up with a double dose of gender and cultural messages, sometimes confusingly at odds with each other. Without guides or models of how to be our hyphenated selves, we experimented, discarded, made mistakes, conferred with each other. And so, by trial and error and the seat of my pants (some of them hanging in this very closet), I worked my way through selves I discovered I could be, some brief, some destined to become a core part of me.

I don't regret any of these choices. They were the only options I thought I had at that moment in time. But finally at fifty, it was time to release them. I would no longer dress to appeal to the male gaze that was no longer turning my way anyhow. From now on, I would wear only the clothes I felt comfortable in, ones that weren't meant to improve, disguise, or minimize my "bad" features, make me look like an airbrushed, bogus me. As a dozen or more outfits went into a box for the local secondhand shop, I felt a mess of emotions, from death throes and pangs of nevermore to a thrilling curiosity about what lay ahead now that a half century of living was over.

For this watershed birthday, I wanted to mark the passage with something more significant than just cleaning out my closet. I come from a Latin culture steeped in custom and ceremony. "We are a ritual people," Octavio Paz once remarked. We love our fiestas and festivals, a way to stop the flow of time and commemorate an occasion. One Latina friend threw herself a cincuentañera when she turned fifty, an older-life version of our traditional quinceañera celebrating a young girl's symbolic arrival into womanhood. Actually, the first rite of passage for a female in the DR of my childhood was when she was born, the doctor would pierce her ears. This was so automatic, Mami told me, that you had to specify if you did *not* want your baby's ears to be touched. And so, after cleaning out my closet, I headed downtown to a little notions shop where a lot of the local teens had their ears pierced, and I got a second piercing above the ones I'd had since the day I was born.

"What for?" my husband wanted to know.

I had been pierced at birth, marking my entry into femalehood as understood and mandated by others. This piercing was for a second birth: I was being reborn as the woman I wanted to be, no hiding, no apologies. (I recently heard Jane Fonda say one of the lessons she's finally learned at eighty-five is "*No* is a complete sentence.") "I'm being born again," I told my husband, not as in "giving myself to Jesus," but giving myself to Julia. My life would now be lived, not by reflection or custom or committee (who others wanted me to be) but by that most illusory of creatures, me.

The afterlife of my menopause had begun.

The passage was not all smooth sailing. For one thing, that would not be true to who I am. Smooth sailing is a rare setting on my internal weather app. Menopause was no different. Granted, I was lucky: I did not experience the physical turbulence of two of my sisters and of many cousins and friends: hot flashes, insomnia, heart palpitations, brain fog. ("I had to go to bed with an ice pack," one of my sisters confessed, and when that wasn't enough, she slept in the spare bedroom her grown daughter had vacated, with the air conditioner blasting, even in winter.) I did, however, experience psychic and emotional turbulence. I had to finally make peace with the fact that I would never have a child. The timing had never seemed right. I wasn't settled in a stable marriage until my forties. My husband, Bill, already had two teenage daughters and did not relish the idea of another child, which would require undoing a vasectomy he'd had over a decade ago. Family dynamics were complicated. It was tricky enough starting a new family of four, without immediately adding a fifth. And I was busy launching my career as a teacher and writer, traveling and touring with my books. From time to time, I suffered bouts of indecision, often triggered by a heedless remark. One cringe comment came from a male colleague who described childless female writers (Jane Austen, Emily Dickinson, George Eliot) as committing "genetic suicide." Now, at fifty, the possibility I always held out that maybe one day, quizás, quién sabe, I might bear a child, was gone. A firm period at the end of my periods. I had erased the future of me.

Along with that erasure, there were others. More and more, the young and not so young men and women looked over my shoulder at the new arrivals in the field of time. Aging was not something to celebrate, or even acknowledge. Instead, the consumer culture encouraged me to buy products and services and B.S. ("Fifty is the new thirty," etc.) to hide my age, as if it were a source of shame. One night at dinner a friend of my granddaughter alluded to my age and immediately clapped her hand over her mouth, mortified. "I'm so sorry," she apologized, "I didn't mean to call you old."

"Old is all right," I assured her. How disheartening to think that this young woman was dreading this stage of life, where she was bound if she lived long enough, but I was glad that I could provide a positive model of an "old" person at home in her weathered body and at ease with herself.

Positive role models were rare when I was going through menopause twenty-five years ago. Older women were not given much visibility except in commercials for medications or in sitcoms where the caricature of the old bag or loopy mother-in-law triggered canned laughter.

In my Dominican culture, elders fared better. Not that older women ever talked about this passage, just as they didn't talk about any other sexual matters, except in generalities and euphemisms: becoming a señorita (code for getting your menses), doing your duty by your husband (having married sex—any other kind was taboo), *dando a luz* (giving to the light, certainly a glorified way to describe the messy labor of giving birth). Menopause was no different. "*Los calores,*" one aunt called it, like the heat waves of summer, or "*el cambio,*" the change. They fanned themselves vigorously, slept poorly, suffered in silence and said one more rosary. Many were widows, dressed in drab luto for the rest of their lives as a sign of their devotion to the memory of their husbands. This was not quite like being thrown in the pyre with your just-deceased spouse, but it was death to any sexual self: The adventures of the flesh were over. Instead, these older women turned their attention to religious matters, attending daily mass, volunteering in church activities, taking up charity work and the care of family members, especially grandchildren. Abuelas do hold a venerable and vital place in our culture. This helps with the transition, for sure.

But none of these Old or New World models were viable or appealing. I had to find my own elder clan for guidance, muses to help me get wherever I was going.

One of the reliable places I go to for guidance is stories. At certain stages in my life, one or another story or poem or song will become important to me. I call these "stories to steer by," a kind of narrative GPS, string for the labyrinth. They don't give me specific instructions or prepackaged popular "truths." They are more reminders of the things I don't want to discard along with those past selves and outfits—what Stanley Kunitz in his wonderful poem, "The Layers," calls "some principle of being [which] abides." These stories and poems have changed over time, depending on where I am in my own life and what I need to focus on going forward.

When we arrived in the USA and into English, I became a reader, not just out of love of narrative, but out of a pressing need to understand my new culture and country: Nancy Drew mysteries, *Little Women*, stories with feisty girls who were smart, resilient problem-solvers who followed their passions.

Their fabricated worlds became the spaces where I lived most intensely; they were my companions, the soulmates I turned to for direction and nurture.

Over the years, the narratives I chose—or did they choose me?—were ones that helped me make meaning and reframed each new stage in my life. As I aged, I read anything I could find where the protagonist was an older woman. Not just fiction, either. Biographies of artists and their work in old age. "The late style," Edward Said called it in his book on the subject that— no surprise—deals mostly with male writers and musicians. I needed authors who would do for menopause and old age what Judy Blume had done for menses and adolescence—by exploring this significant upheaval in a female body and life, which affects half of the population. "OLD WOMEN ARE YOUR FUTURE," read a poster at a recent women's march attended by The Old Women's Project, an activist group of female elders based in San Diego. The stories we tell ourselves about menopause and aging will determine not just our future but the future of girls coming after us, like my granddaughter and her friend.

Navigating by narrative is not just a literary bias. It's in our DNA, as I discovered in reading *Songlines*, Bruce Chatwin's account of Aboriginal cosmology and lore. Chatwin tells of tribes on the northwest coast of America that lived half on the islands and half on the mainland. They would travel over the sea and navigate their canoes up the current from California to the Bering Strait, which they called Klin Otto. The navigators were priestesses. The words of this old woman represent a tradition about fifteen thousand years old.

Everythin' we ever knew about the movement of the sea was preserved in the verses of a song. For thousands of years, we went where we wanted and came home safe, because of the song. On clear nights we had the stars to guide us, and in the fog we had the streams and the creeks of the sea, the streams and creeks that flow into and become Klin Otto...

There was a song for goin' to China and a song for goin' to Japan, a song for the big island and a song for the smaller one. All she had to know was the song and she knew where she was. To get back, she just sang the song in reverse.

It still gives me goose bumps to think that all along I've been following an ancient female-centered tradition of using songs to steer by. And more meaningful now than ever, those piloting tellers were old women.

What are the stories that might provide us with nourishment, physical, mental, emotional, spiritual, at this stage of our lives? Working, as women are wont to do, in circles and cycles rather than hierarchies from the top down, communally, not singly, we need to collect ourselves and tell the stories we've lived and found useful, talismanic narratives to keep us safe and bring us home to ourselves. "The time of the lone wolf is over," a message from Hopi Elders reminded us at the dawn of the new millennium. "Gather yourselves...We are the ones we have been waiting for."

And so for the remainder of this journey, in the guise of one of those old priestesses, I want to share a few of the stories and poems that have helped me navigate my way and make meaning of my mid-to-later life as a woman: the perimenopausal stage, menopause itself, and this last stage I call the afterlife of menopause, which is where I live now.

The years leading up to my fiftieth birthday had been exhausting as I drove myself to secure a place at what Langston Hughes in his poem, "I, too, Sing America," called the big table of Literature. (Meanwhile, he and his fellow writers of color were relegated to the kitchen of minor writers.) It seemed to have taken "forever" to get there! At forty-one, after twenty-plus years of writing and dozens of rejections, I finally published my first novel. Nine years later, when I turned fifty, I had written eight more books, traveled on tours promoting them, while also teaching my college courses, earning tenure, judging contests, blurbing books, sitting on panels, writing short pieces and op-eds on the topic du jour—all the cutting ribbon stuff you do as an aspiring writer. (I had yet to get the memo about *No* being a complete sentence.)

I shake my head now with weary compassion for that little racehorse woman who couldn't stop and take care of herself. At one Q & A after a reading in Denver or maybe Miami or Chicago or San Francisco, a member of the audience asked me to describe my writing process. "I just try to stay one sentence ahead of the furies," I replied. The furies were the naysayers, external *and* internal, who for two-plus decades had denied me my literary green card. I was an immigrant whose English wasn't even her first language—how could I presume I belonged on this country's bookshelves? Now that I had been allowed "in," I worried that if I stopped and took the breather everyone kept urging me to take—while also asking me to come deliver the keynote at their conference or visit their son's English class—I would be deported back to the anonymous margins.

The go-to story of those years was that of Scheherazade of *The Arabian Nights*. Ever since reading that book as a child, I had been enthralled by this bold, clever girl who had saved her life and the lives of all the women in the kingdom by telling stories that mesmerized the misogynist sultan. I wanted to be that storyteller, and by writing and publishing and garnering recognition and awards, I had become that girl who survived and transformed the sultans/furies/editors/naysayers who had once dismissed me.

Except, I wasn't a girl anymore. My body began showing the wear and tear. I lost weight and with that my periods, slept poorly, dosed myself with antidepressants and melatonin. I did have a few wake-up calls: a scary episode of misdiagnosed throat cancer, asthma attacks, acid reflux that made me lose my voice. My poor body was signaling: Let me out of here! But as a female, I had learned to subdue the needs of my body to whatever was required of me. My parents' fierce immigrant work ethic added fuel to the fire in my belly. We could never let down our guard or lower our standards. We had to show "them" we deserved to stay here. In la familia's operating system, there was no such thing as a pause-to-rest button.

In my late forties, a part of the Scheherazade story I had side-lined became more compelling. Scheherazade had saved not just herself with her storytelling but all the women in the king-dom. As a published author I was now in a position to advocate for others. (A key steering mantra of those years was Toni Mor-rison's remark that "the function of freedom is to free someone else.") I'd always thought of myself as a reluctant activist—the excuse had been that no one listens to me anyhow—but now they were listening and I had to speak out. The writing and publication of my second novel based on the lives of three rev-olutionary sisters in the Dominican Republic who had been eliminated by the dictator further politicized me. Increasingly, after its publication, I was invited to speak out against human rights abuses and violence against women as well as the ongo-ing marginalization of writers of color. In the end, my own words had pulled me into activism.

Several real-life "priestesses" mused and mentored me. My warrior-woman agent/angel, Susan Bergholz, a petite woman with outsized courage, assembled a pack of us—we called our-selves Las Girlfriends, abriendo caminos, kicking ass. I've always been braver when accompanied by sisters, and my posse of com-pañeras led by Susan breathed grit into me, Sandra Cisneros, Ana Castillo, Denise Chavez, Helena María Viramontes, Cherríe Moraga, among others. Together, we were leveraging our talents and success to open up opportunities for other marginalized sto-rytellers, drowning out the sultan's misogynist can'ts with ¡Sí se puede! Yes, we can!

Another unlikely priestess turned out to be my mother. In

her early fifties Mami began volunteering at the Dominican Republic mission at the United Nations, working late hours, attending meetings, writing up the notes, doing the maintenance cleaning because, as she told me by way of explanation when I asked why she was carrying paper towels and a bottle of Fantastic in her briefcase, "We're a poor country. Why spend money on cleaning when we can do it ourselves?" Her work habits made her indispensable at the mission. When a new administration came into power back home, Mami was assigned a full-time post as *alternate* ambassador—she was a woman, after all, a male was picked as the ambassador. Her focus became the Third Committee, where she campaigned for the human rights of elders and women and children around the world. She succeeded in getting the General Assembly to pass The Principles of Older Persons as well as to proclaim an annual Day of Older Persons, earning the informal title among her colleagues of "the ambassador on aging." Along with others in the Dominican mission, she proposed the UN set aside a day for the elimination of violence against women: November 25, the day of the murder of the sisters I had written about in my historical novel, *In the Time of the Butterflies.*

My sisters and I were dumbfounded. Mami?! Really?! Mami, who was always warning of the dire consequences of choosing careers over traditional marriages and motherhood; who had given us the silent treatment for "answering her back" (she was now mouthing off, politely, to world leaders!); who threatened to pull us out of college for protesting against the Vietnam War (Mami was now marching with the Gray Panthers in

Nueva York). Finally midlife our mother had found a canvas large enough for her energy and talents: the whole world. If only she'd found it sooner, my sisters and I commiserated, we would have had a much easier childhood.

This major shift in her life began soon after my mother turned fifty. Only now am I putting it together that Mami had been going through menopause with her bad migraines and insomnia and dragon-lady meltdowns. One of my sisters recently recalled finding birth control pills in Mami's bedside table. When my sister asked about them, Mami burst into tears. "It's not what you think," she sobbed. "Think what?" my sister asked. But Mami wouldn't say. The cultural gag order was firmly in place.

Sometimes she turned that gag order on us. Particularly on her nemesis and namesake, the other Julia. When my first novel was published my mother was ashamed that family secrets would crush her nascent career at the UN. "But it's fiction, Mami!" didn't fly with her. There were too many similarities to our family, and the Mami in the book was not the smart, professional world-class diplomat she was trying to present to the world. She hired a lawyer and threatened to sue me for ruining her career. With persuasion by family and friends, not to mention that her career never suffered from my writing, she dropped the suit and over the years became one of my biggest supporters. But it was rocky there for a while. Often our priestesses do double service as our demons. Mami's training was so ingrained she felt she had "to protect our family name." All the more power to her that she was ultimately able to rise above her conservative upbringing and advocate for women and elders around the world. Instead of hoping I didn't grow up and turn out to be like her, now as I grow old, I hope I have inherited some of her fierce DNA.

In my early postmenopausal years, a downpour of losses began to steadily rain down on me. I had always considered myself lucky in having an extended Dominican family of loving tías, tíos, madrinas, padrinos, providing a buffer between me and the end of me. The problem was when they started going, it was not just one or two significant others, but dozens. Suddenly, it seemed, a whole phalanx of my elders was going down, which included my parents, both of whom I'd been losing for years to dementia. Along with my mood, the color palette in my closet darkened with funeral outfits. The most devastating loss was that of my sister, whom I adored. I didn't think I could survive her suicide. It seemed most of the people I loved were on the other side. Why not join them?

Along with everything else, stories lost their luster, their power to comfort and guide me. So much complicated, frivolous narrative noise! I couldn't get engaged in reading or writing. That was the scariest part: I had lost my purchase on words. I was mute with grief.

During this time I would often go to the college library and sit by a series of prints by the artist Sabra Field, displayed on a stretch of wall. Her Demeter Suite depicted the myth of Demeter, who loses her daughter Persephone to the underworld. In her grief, Demeter, goddess of the harvest, blasts the earth with endless winter. She, too, could not get over the loss of someone she loved. This woman was a kindred spirit. I felt accompanied.

The penultimate print showed Demeter reunited with her daughter. Persephone has been allowed to come back for a spell before she has to return to the underworld. Spring returns to the earth, flowers grow, fields turn golden with grain. I stroked that framed print as if hope were contagious.

This story kept a pilot light burning in me. In its glow my spirits began to revive. The story of Demeter helped me reframe my experience. I was no longer immortal—that feeling in youth that life is inexhaustible and energy boundless. Going forward, my body would experience little deaths, as I reached the expiration dates of any number of body parts, hopefully the replaceable ones. But spring would return. "And now in age I bud again," writes the poet, George Herbert, in "The Flower," one of the talismanic poems of this stage of my life. "After so many deaths I live and write; / I once more smell the dew and rain / and relish versing."

I ended up contacting Sabra Field. She confided that she had recently lost her husband. She, too, was in mourning. We decided to work together on a picture book about grief "for children of all ages." I began writing again.

"Practice resurrection," Wendell Berry advises in another favorite poem of this stage of my life. "Be joyful—though you have considered all the facts." Keeping our spirits burning bright is the challenge of this late stage in life—a gift we elders can give to ourselves and others: a sense of recurring possibilities, joy springing up from the ashes, but also acceptance of losses, including our own eventual demise. "All of us go down to the dust," the Anglican burial prayer reminds us—and I have been to more of these services lately than I can count—"yet even at the grave we make our song, Alleluia, Alleluia, Alleluia."

This ushers in the current stage of my journey in this female body that has been and seen and done so much. "There is a crack…in everything that's how the light gets in," Leonard Cohen sings in his song, "Anthem." Old age's wrinkles and scars provide plenty of cracks if we don't try to patch them up and pretend they are not there. And that light is critical as night falls and the dark sets in.

Living in the afterlife of menopause, I practice daily resurrections, I make my song. Instead of guides, I search out companion priestesses. The older the better. (Two of my closest friends are ten and eleven years older than I am.) Of course, I'm energized and charmed by the beautiful vibrancy of the young, but I often find myself missing some of the rich layers that texture and deepen interactions.

The stories I steer by these days are songs of love, the agape kind, which has a more widespread root system than Eros. The green of spring fades—"my salad days," Shakespeare's Cleopatra calls them—but this dead vegetation provides necessary nourishment for the seeds buried in the soil. I like the idea of being compost. Being of use. Nurturing the new generations. More and more I feel deeply connected to the earth and its rhythms, more and more committed to its regeneration from the wounds I've participated in inflicting. In Hopi traditions when an elder is ordained to a higher religious order, the earth and all living things are placed in her hands. She is now the parent and grandparent of all life on earth. My favorite story to steer by these days is about a woman who has been reaching for the stars all her life. Finally as an old woman she touches them. At which point Father Sky looks at her and asks, "How'd you get to be so tall?" She answers, "I'm standing on a lot of shoulders."

I am taller than I would be for all the shoulders I have stood on, and growing taller as I offer my shoulders to the young generations whose turn it is to reach for whatever star they've chosen to steer by.

This is what the afterlife of menopause looks like from the altitude of gratitude.

Alleluia! Alleluia! Alleluia!

SHE-DANDY

By Darcey Steinke

I recognize her immediately. Upwards of seventy, gray hair cut close to her head, fitted pants above brown leather boots, the lavender sweater vest over a white blouse open at the neck to show an amulet resting on her chiseled clavicle. In her hands, a well-worn paperback, which she less reads than falls into.

On my way to the dentist, I spot another sitting at an out-door cafe. Braids piled high on her head, she is resplendent in her long black floral dress, large, crème-colored flowers coming out of the dark, a small glittery scarf tied at her neck. She wears large-frame sunglasses and red lipstick.

There are also the many she-dandys on the down low, the lady with the purple puffer jacket and gray ponytail chasing her grandson down the street, and the woman outside the hospital leaning into a bronze-topped cane in her frayed camel hair coat.

In 2022 I happened on an essay by the poet Lisa Robertson. In Robertson's telling the she-dandy demonstrates with her body that the only real worthiness is adding to human fragility. Not pretending it does not exist. Who wouldn't want to revel in the power of being so close to oblivion? I've always wanted to transcend my linear existence and connect to the eternal. But it's human to feel trapped in this corporeal envelope, and I, too, have at times tried to prop up an earlier self. Not long ago I was going to dinner at the apartment of a man I use to have a crush on. We had never dated but long ago, before he was married, he had told me that he wanted to. That this charge had existed called up a former self, one worried about looking desirable.

I began to fixate on what to wear. *Should I wear a dress, instead of my usual pants and sweatshirts?* I have to confess—I know judging others is wrong—but there have been times I've been angry with women who pretend not to be aging. I had grown to find it offensive to those of us who are involved in the difficult work of decomposition. But now, I was on that other side. *Should I go out to the drugstore and buy makeup, which I no longer used, to get that promised youthful effect?*

At the time, I was in Paris doing research for a new book, and between visits to Le Musée des Moulages—a wax museum devoted to skin disease—and another that held old surgery equipment, I shopped. I envisioned myself in a dress, that without making me look ridiculous, would bring back the illusion of freshness. I eventually found the dress, green, with an empire waist and a long flowing skirt to the floor. In the dressing room mirror I appraised myself. From the neck down, covered in green silk there was no way to know I was sixty-one, but from the neck up was another story. My face is no longer strictly female. I am androgynous now, as well as wrinkled with crinkly under eyes, heavy cheeks that create indentions around my mouth, and a Y-shaped fissure in my forehead.

Soon, the night of the dinner arrived, and I tried on the dress. Looking at myself in the mirror, I remember my mother, even at age thirty, crying to my father that she didn't want to get old, and how as a teenager, I had obsessed on the faint lines under my eyes. Now I was actually old. Was the dress trying too hard? *What gives me the right, at my age, to ornament myself?* I thought.

One part of me swiftly answered myself back: *All women my age, or any age, should be able to wear whatever the fuck we want.* But before I know it, I am thinking of Miss Havisham in her ratty wedding dress. I am picturing Blanche DuBois with her thick foundation, trying to trick a man into accepting her ruse of youth and inexperience. I also know these depictions were created by men. And looking back, I can see: My unease with the green dress wasn't shame. I was uncomfortable in performing a version of my femininity out of sync with who I was. Of all the many things I've learned from trans people, the most inspirational is that no matter the sex we are assigned at birth, we each have the right to present ourselves how we feel on the inside. In the end I didn't wear the dress, but instead put together an outfit that better represents my post-reproductive identity: white leather pants, a Simone de Beauvoir T-shirt, and a pair of bright orange Hokas.

All my adult life I've worried about aging. I bought firming

mud masks and special face creams. But it wasn't until menopause that I truly understood I would have to change. Ten years
ago, at fifty-one, I no longer bled monthly, and I suffered episodes of panic and suffocating heat. Unable to sleep, I walked
room to room in my Brooklyn house in the darkest hours of the
night. Those first awful months found me standing before the
window and crying out *Help me!* to the bright, clueless moon.
My mother had recently died, so could neither advise nor support me.

When I planned her service, I had chosen not to see my
mother's dead body, which resided in the funeral home morgue,
and chose a closed casket. Looking back, I see cowardice. I was
afraid of catching death from her. She was completely dead,
only a part of me was. But I was discovering that even a little
deadness was disorienting.

I had always dismissed the implication that just because
women's bodies can carry babies, every monthly cycle that does
not lead to pregnancy makes us feel (even if we do not want a
child) sad, lost, empty. Now I did feel, with every hot flash, that
my old self was burning off, creating internal and external vacu-
ums. This new emptiness was different from earlier variations,
heartache's desperation, depression's gray listlessness, grief's
heavy introspection. It carried not only a chaotic emotional
state, but also the intimation of fleshy collapse.

When I visited my doctor, a woman a little older than
myself, complaining of sudden heat, sleeplessness, pain during
intercourse—she did not suggest I might be moving into menopause. I was left, like so many of us, to google it out by myself.

What I found made me furious. A medical world describing my transition as a disease. On medical websites I read terms for the menopausal body, sagging breasts, geriatric ovaries, shrunken vulva, shriveled uterus. It seemed less descriptive than mean. Multiple humor sites made jokes about my unstable emotions, my sweatiness, my chin hairs, my dried-up cunt.

As a writer, I tried to find books that would help me understand. There were medical texts and a few memoirs, in both, after a period of suffering, hormones were offered as "the cure" for menopausal symptoms. Certainly, no book dealt with the metaphysical aspects of what I was going through, or the sensation that I was split, a failing body and a soul struggling to get out.

⁓

Oddly, the hero of *Flash Count Diary*, the book I would eventually write about menopause, was not me, but a 105-year-old killer whale named J2, and nicknamed Granny. After menopause at around 45, older female orcas begin to lead their pods. They are upfront in the search for salmon; they help younger whales with mating rituals; and they support adolescent and pregnant members of their pods, by swimming near them, giving advice and corralling fish for them to eat.

Through the study of Granny's pod and other orcas that live in the Salish Sea off Washington State, scientists have posited out a possible reason for menopause, a life process that had previously confused them. Menopause, they speculated, allowed not just whales but also humans in their earliest pre-human hunter-gatherer phase to split into two distinct groups: one to do the important work of birthing and raising children—and the older group, to lead.

I got to see Granny once on a kayak trip out in the Salish Sea. I recognized her by the notch I had seen in pictures of her dorsal fin. Her large shining body overwhelmed me. Till then I could not believe in the goddess. To me the idea of a female deity was sentimental, overly positive, new age, depleted of any alive-meaning and the progenitor of a lot of terrible art, but J2 was the OG, otherly, smelly, powerful, ridiculously awake. The contact high of seeing her led me through the writing of my book, and the years of my own transition. Our exchange was not soft focus, not a moment of human-creature bonding as one some-times reads between a rich lady and her elephant. No. Her eye was large, dark, and censorious. I was in the presence of wild-ness, provocative and enigmatic.

Killer whales are crazy smart, their brains are three times as large as humans, and contain spindle cells, tissue associated with empathy. Did she sense how I projected all my hopes for my own later years onto her? Maybe J2's concerns were strictly ecological. She surely knew that I was human and associated humans with the fishing boats that over-fish salmon, and the dams that block salmon runs, and the massive container ships that mess up her and her pod's echolocation. But over the years, since the encounter, I've wondered if J2 might have also rec-ognized me as another aging female. Who knows, maybe that strange leering eyeball, like a censorious grapefruit, was saying *deal with your own fucking self.*

Is it even possible to accept your body's decay? Clearly it's work that takes a while, it can't be accomplished at a weekend yoga retreat or by writing oneself letters of affirmation, or making gratitude lists. I know because as my body started slowly to break, I tried all of these. At fifty-seven I herniated a disc in my back. The strongest pain reliever I was given while I tried to resolve the issue with physical therapy was Tylenol. I took them by the handful and drank one glass of rosé after another. After nine months of agony, of feeling like a broken marionette, I had successful back surgery. Not long into my recovery, I cracked a tooth and when it was pulled, a hole ripped in my sinus. Another period of pain, followed by sinus surgery. These ruptures were scary but it wasn't until the chest pain that I started to really freak out.

I had the heart MRI in an old office building in midtown and by the time I got off the subway in Brooklyn, I already had an email with my results. My left coronary artery was 66 percent blocked and I was in the eighty-seventh percentile for heart diseases for my age group. Days followed when I felt I was under a bell jar, not able to understand what people said to me and terrified of every twinge or tightness in my chest. Was my slight cough just allergies or a sign of congestive heart failure? And maybe those episodes of intense pressure at my sternum weren't indigestion after all. The worst time was at night when I watched YouTube videos of echo cardiograms and listened to what a normal left artery sounded like, oil moving smoothly through a metal pipe—versus the glub, glub, glub of a blocked one. I understood that my old way of treating life and death like two distinct countries would no longer work, I would need now to integrate the immaterial with the material. My mother had died of a heart attack caused by coronary artery disease at seventy: How much time would I have left?

—

Urgently, I began searching out she-dandys. Women who had worked to integrate, in their own bodies, the living and the dead. "Ah my God, what is it that we love," wrote one of my favorite writers, Djuna Barnes, "this flesh laid on us like a wrinkled glove?" In her "Book of Repulsive Women," Barnes embraces her body's decay. Sometimes it's hard to tell, whether the bodies she is writing about are dead or alive. In the poem "The Flying Corpse," a cadaver continues to grow. "Over the body and the quiet head / Like stately ferns above an austere tomb, / Soft hairs blow; and beneath her armpits bloom." Her poem suggests that death might not be the end, that there might be a forever channel inside nature.

Even as a young reporter in New York City, Barnes used her body to test mortality and connect with others. In one 1913 article for the *Brooklyn Daily Eagle*, she agreed to be force-fed in solidarity with the imprisoned British suffragettes. As Barnes comes out of the haze of tranquilizers and the feeding tube is removed from her throat, she is wobbly, only half animal. "It was over. I stand up, swaying in the returning light, I had shared the greatest experience of the bravest of my sex."

Barnes died in 1982 at the age of ninety. In her last years she lived as a recluse in a one-room apartment on Patchin Place in the West Village. I don't know if she ever accepted her own decay. It hardly matters though because her struggle remains so vivid. When I pass her apartment on my way to teach my NYU class, I feel its charge.

—

I look for guidance in coming to terms with my mortality in even the most mundane places. On my kitchen counter inside my compost bin, vegetable scrapes rot. They send up a thick putrid smell and attract fruit flies. On Sunday mornings I carry this bucket to a station near Prospect Park, where I dump the weeping produce into a larger bin where it gets mixed with my neighbors'. This ritual, over the years, has gained meaning. I use to sit in a pew on Sundays, subscribing to a theology of supernatural renewal. Now my compost brings me up close to the earth's actual regeneration. In his poem praising compost, Walt Whitman felt it was a process, unlike the afterlife, that one could count on. "This is no cheat this transparent green-wash." He compares rot to romantic love, naming the way the earth calls us back to itself as "amorous."

—

I finally followed my fascination to the real thing. In January 2023 I drove out to Pennsylvania to see a dead body. The anatomy professor who invited me told me that his students had just dissected the cadavers' chests and that I should hurry before the heart and other organs dried out. The dissection room of the medical school was white and silver, the dozen corpses lay in straight lines on gurneys. There was a big metal sink where we washed our hands and put on plastic gloves. The bodies were covered in blue towels soaked in a concoction of Pine-Sol and fabric-softener and each was covered by a thick sheet of clear plastic.

The professor, a man in his early seventies with shaggy gray hair and a small gold earring, wears a pink calico shirt. He lifts the plastic, the blue towels, then carefully opens the strange leathery cabinet of the cadaver's chest. I can see the rib cage, which he removes: the lungs, milky and beautiful, and finally the heart, pinkish gray and larger than I expected. He lifts it out from where it has been severed from its arteries and connective tissue and hands it to me. It is heavy, with an interesting weight, like a glass paperweight.

I ask him to point out the left artery, nicknamed the widow maker, which in my pump is blocked. A delicate fleshy tube, like an earthworm, that clings to the heart surface. The professor goes on to show me the various chambers, each with a tiny door cut out by the students, that lets me see the interior valves and muscles. Setting the heart back into its place in the body, he pulls the towel down further to show me the rest of the chest cavity of this very small, very dead, woman. The intestines, her kidneys, he has me touch the hard cancer cells inside her pancreas. Once the intestines have been lifted, I see the colon and at the bottom of the pelvis, what looks like a deflated gray balloon, attached on either side to a bit of dirty string and at each end a chickpea: the uterus, fallopian tubes, and ovaries.

I assumed it would be profound to see the heart, the organ that might one day kill me. But what affected me more was the reproductive organs. Before the cadaver, I imagined the womb backlit and glorious. A glowing fetus inside, its aura not unlike the sparkle from the Milky Way. So different from the little bit of chicken skin the professor pointed out as the atrophied uterus.

—

Sometimes I wonder, if I'd witnessed my mother's dead body, would I understand death better? Maybe seeing the lifeless body I came out of would have helped me to accept my own demise? That option is long gone. After her funeral, my mother was cremated and her ashes buried. So I continue to look for help, as I always do, in books.

In *Change of Life,* psychoanalyst Ann Mankowitz helps her patient Rachel move past menopause. Rachel is fifty-one, married with three grown children, though any domestic safety she once felt has evaporated. Rachel dreams of a burnt-out house, charred fetuses hanging from the black rafters. "It's me," Rachel tells Mankowitz, "my insides, but not just that, my past life, my children, that whole way of life ended forever."

In her dream, the front wall of the house has burned off and Rachel can see inside. "In a bedroom, on a large double bed, lies a woman, not old, not young... she gives the appearance of fullness, smoothness, and maturity. She could be alive and asleep but I know she is dead…feelings of inexpressible sadness and pity come over me." For several sessions, Rachel struggles. How will she move forward now that she is dead? Mankowitz reports a breakthrough when her patient reinterprets an odd detail, the woman was "green," not rotting, but with a skin tone akin to an early spring leaf.

Is it even possible for an aging woman to *green*? To be plant-like? The philosopher Michael Marder writes in his book, *Plant Thinking*, that to green is to "take an apprenticeship in non-verbal language." Plants' main project is to extend themselves further into space, "to grow." Their alertness is not like human alertness, he insists, which is summoned by danger and death. The plant instead pays attention in its silent meditation "to the element of continuity."

The greenness I seek is about eternity not youth. A flower farmer recently told me how it makes her angry that people associate flowers with the young. "The flowering plant is at the end of its life cycle. A flower is a grand old lady, not a prepubescent bud." The flower, in other words, is a she-dandy.

⁓

In July I get invited to read at Willow Wisp, an organic farm in Damascus, Pennsylvania. After trying on pants and various tops, I decide on the Paris dress. As I climb up onto the outdoor stage in view of a large compost pile, I realize my dress, like a giant leaf, grows out from a memory of my mother when I was seven or eight. Her dress was made of smooth green satin, with a little fitted jacket she held over her pale arm. In the dress, my mother was a woman but also more than a woman. Her meaning expanded, overflowing her familiar form. What I really want, I now understand, is not fertility but fecundity, a process I can be part of even when, like my mother, I am dead. Outside the tent it started to rain, a soft sound on the canvas. I look over the crowd, hold up the typed pages of my new book and open my mouth, each sentence as I read, unfurls like a vine moving out toward the light.

LATE, BLOOMING

By Roxane Gay

Recently, my father sent me a picture of my cousin Ariane's christening. In it, I was fourteen or so, her godmother. Another cousin was her godfather. We were all very young. We stood with the priest around the baptismal font, in our baptismal finery. Ariane was screaming her tiny, adorable head off in the priest's arms. At first, I didn't recognize myself in the photo. I remembered myself as much bigger. For nearly two years, I had been gaining weight and no one understood why. I knew, of course. I had made a choice to build a wall of flesh around myself, to make myself safe after being desperately unsafe. My family was panicked. They immediately shifted into overreaction, trying to solve the problem of my body but my body was not actually a problem, at least not to me.

That's why, in the decades since, I am impossibly large in my recollections. That's how extravagantly the people around me reacted to my changing body. The picture, though, seeing it so many years later, was startling. It was evidence that the story I told myself for so long—a story architected by people who meant well but caused harm nonetheless—was not the truth. Certainly, I looked awkward because I was wearing a cream-colored, satiny dress with boxy shoulders and I hated wearing dresses. They looked terrible on me, like I was playing dress-up with a very different girl's wardrobe. I sported a weird haircut because I had no sense of style yet. I simply wanted to be invisible. My body was incidental, a vessel for my fractured mind. But, in reality, I was cute. I had a baby face. I was not fat, at all. So many years later, in a much larger body, I would love to be that size again. I would revel in it. And I would love to have recognized, back then, that there was nothing wrong with me at any size.

—

I am my father's only daughter and while my brothers and I were each our parents' favorites in different ways, I am his favorite. He had dreams for me as his only daughter, his American girl, and most of those dreams conflicted with who I actually was. This happens between parents and children. Even though he never explicitly articulated his dreams I knew he wanted me to be girly and popular. Maybe he wanted me to be a cheerleader, bright and bubbly, pretty in pink. Instead, he got a shy, quiet introvert who spent most of her time with her head in a book. This wasn't necessarily a bad thing and he encouraged my reading and eventually, my writing. But as the only girl with two brothers, I was far more inclined to be something of a tomboy. I eschewed overly feminine things, and while people assumed it was because I was a tomboy, that wasn't really the case. I eschewed anything that would bring attention to myself. I took comfort in oversized shirts and sweaters, baggy pants, anything that would shroud my ever-expanding body.

During the years when I was supposed to be taking an interest in boys, going on dates, maybe embarking on a sweet relationship with a first love, there was no one in my vicinity who was even remotely interested. I had crushes that were, mostly, silly affectations because I felt like I was supposed to have a crush and yearn dramatically. If I doodled some boy's name on my notebook and drew hearts while I gazed into the distance, daydreaming, maybe I would become a real girl. Unfortunately, I was never that good at doing what was expected of me when it came to social graces.

What my real life lacked, I more than compensated for with my imagination. In truth, I hated boys—their bravado and the tangy smell they carried in their skin. I hated their loud voices and growing muscles and how easily they took up space as if it was their due. But I wanted to be like the other girls, the normal girls. I wanted boys to want me before I understood that really, I wanted girls to want me. I wanted to wear a letterman jacket, have a boy hold my hand, ask me out on a date, recognize that I was a girl too, with a hungry girl heart. I succeeded in my desire to be invisible. The attention I did get from boys and then men was always furtive, often sleazy, and very transactional. They took and I gave and I told myself it was enough.

—

When you are fat in a fat-phobic world, you tend to live in a pecu-
liar state of longing, a state of perpetual anticipation, making
yourself promises about all the things you will do when.

W

   h

      e

         n

            W

               h

                  e

                     n

                        W

                           h

                             e

                               n

You plan your life around the bounty that awaits when you
lose enough weight to find a loving partner, to get a good job, to
travel abroad, to visit parents without intense anxiety, to make
everyone happy, to make yourself happy. This fraught limbo is
how I lived through my teens, my twenties, my thirties. Decades
of waiting go by until you reach middle age and are forced to ask
yourself, "When will I really start living?" Even once I started
to embrace body neutrality in my forties, I nurtured this stasis,
as if life would only truly begin when I was the right size and
what a short life it would be. I wasted so much time I will never
get back. There was never going to be a right size so long as I

believed I was the problem. And oh, how I believed that, into the marrow of my bones. I couldn't believe otherwise no matter how hard I tried.

As women, we are told relentlessly, in so many different ways, that youth and beauty and thinness are currency. It is how we communicate our value to the world. As we age, that currency becomes less powerful and then, we simply fade from relevance, left, hopefully, in peace to enjoy our dotage. If you don't meet the standards of conventional attraction, your currency is less powerful. And when you are fat, when you inhabit an unruly body, you have no currency at all. I didn't always know this but once I learned, I was a perfect student.

For years, I also told myself that when I emerged from this stasis, when I was the right size, I would finally be a real woman, where a real woman was thin, beautiful, desired—someone who had currency, someone who would be able to enjoy womanly things, be seen as and treated like a woman, even if I also had to deal with the challenges of womanhood with which most other women contend.

I had all these yearnings, but I was also furious with myself for wanting things that intellectually, at least, I found reductive, problematic, or misogynistic. That's the terrible bind of body tyranny. We are taught to want the things that harm us most.

What I really mean is that I always hoped to be treated with care, with tenderness. I hoped people might recognize I could be as delicate as I am strong. I hoped people might truly see me. But fatness renders women genderless or, at least, that has been my experience of fatness. Fatness renders women not only invisible but also inconvenient, always in the way, always taking up too much space. People will stare too hard, make their snide little comments, sigh with impatience when I am walking too slowly, make it clear in one way or another that for them, my body is a problem, and a serious one at that.

Men have treated me like one of the guys, a person so far beyond the reach of their desires as to be just like them. Women have treated me like one of the guys, a person so far beyond their understanding of womanhood as to be an entirely different species.

All these years, I thought I still had time to enjoy what were supposed to be the best years of my life. I thought I still had time to be a woman. And then, year by year, many of the things I wanted or at least thought I wanted for myself, all that possibility fell away. This is who I am, this is the body I am living in, there is a lot of life left to live, but there are certain experiences I will never have.

In some ways, I never got the chance to be a woman, but this is not a story of regret.

I am fifty years old but I've always been a late bloomer. Even as I stumbled into my teenage years, I was a very young thirteen, fourteen, even fifteen. I got my period later than most girls. I was at boarding school and too shy and self-conscious to ask my mom for guidance, so I went to the Woolworth's in town and browsed the "feminine hygiene" aisle for a very long time, carefully reading the packages of menstrual pads and tampons. It all seemed awkward and uncomfortable. When I got back to my dorm with a box of tampons, I hid in a bathroom stall and pored over the folded instructions several times. This was before You-Tube and Wikipedia. There were no online forums to consult for advice on how to actually use a tampon. It never crossed my mind to ask my mother, who was rather hands off when it came to all things womanhood. The first attempts were awkward and a little painful but eventually, I figured it out and a long, bloody misadventure began.

Even after that, I remained a late bloomer. I didn't grow to my current height until my very late teens, well after everyone assumed I was done growing. I didn't finish graduate school until I was thirty-six. I married in my late forties. For whatever reason, I have always taken a lot of time to become more of myself. And so, when it came to menopause, I expected the worst—having to deal with my period until my late sixties or something equally nightmarish. Once again, I didn't know what to expect. My mother, who went through menopause in her fifties, was pretty circumspect about the experience. She didn't have any of the typical lamentations you might expect. I heard little of hot flashes or all the other bodily changes many women experience. Both of my grandmothers had died many years earlier. Many of my friends were just starting their families in their early forties so menopause was not really on their radar. My wife had gone through menopause years before we met and her experience of it was relatively brief and not terribly disruptive. And, because I had so rarely, throughout my life, been seen or treated as a woman, I sort of assumed that menopause would simply pass me by, the way so many other things had.

The only thing I knew for sure was that with menopause, I would no longer have to deal with my period and that felt like winning the lottery. Every single month, for nearly thirty-five years, I would start to feel despondent and irritable. My breasts became tender. My sex drive was out of control. I was incredibly tired and wanted to sleep all the time. I'd wonder what the hell was going on and start to worry that something might really be wrong. And then, my period would appear and I would realize that all of those weird symptoms were, simply, warning signs. Then, the next month, I started to feel despondent and irritable. My breasts became tender. You get the picture. Sometimes I kept track, first in a paper calendar, later with the Notes app on my phone, and eventually with a series of fertility apps. If I tracked my physical realities assiduously, I might become a real, responsible adult, in command of what little womanhood I had. For decades, I never really learned that my body was always trying to tell me something.

This is to say, I hated my period. I really did. It was inconvenient. I often had really heavy periods. I mean *really* heavy. At times, I worried I would simply bleed out. I wondered where the hell all that blood was coming from. I used an extraordinary number of very big, uncomfortable tampons. I didn't have debilitating cramps or some of the other challenges people with uteruses must contend with, which was, I suppose, a small blessing.

In my mid-forties, my period suddenly became erratic, not that it had ever been particularly disciplined. I would get my period and then it would disappear for a few months. I'd have a delightfully abbreviated period, maybe two days, which absolutely thrilled me. A few months later, I would have a three-week period. Then I would get my period four times in a single month at which point I despaired that I would never, ever stop bleeding. Sometimes, I would start spotting, as if my period was just dipping her toes in the proverbial waters to see if she felt like making a full appearance. As my period came less and less frequently, I started to believe I was finally done with all of that and then yet again she would show up, taunting me, as if to say, "You wish!"

Each time I got my period after three or four months of absence, I was overcome by a wave of frustration that there was no way of knowing which period would be my last. I turned to the internet because my primary physician is a zygote, and I couldn't bring myself to ask her what to expect when I was expecting to never be able to expect again. Dr. Google offered a bewildering range of information about menopause, its symptoms, and what to anticipate. A lot of that information was contradictory and wildly inadequate, a reminder that the medical establishment treats women's bodies as mysterious and unknowable. Whatever goes on in our bodies is none of their concern, unless, of course, we are pregnant, and then for nine months, in certain states, our bodies are not only knowable but legislated, public property.

I knew menopause would happen, but I assumed it wasn't

going to affect me the way it affected other women because I spent so much of my life exiled to the periphery of traditional womanhood. I watched countless depictions of menopause in film and television that showed women worrying about their skin and their libido and hormone levels. I took in all the exaggerated depictions of women in the throes of hot flashes, drenched in sweat, shoving their heads into freezers or sitting in front of oscillating fans looking for respite from an inescapable heat. In *Sex and the City 2*, noted sex enthusiast Samantha Jones brought a small valise of hormones, supplements, and other elixirs she used to stave off the encroachment of "the change" and to "trick my body into thinking it's younger."

When I experienced my first hot flash, it defied everything I had ever imagined. A small fire was burning inside of me and it grew hotter and hotter until I was desperate to extinguish roaring flames I could not reach. When the heat subsided, I never wanted to experience a hot flash ever again. I did, of course, experience more hot flashes, but there was no set pattern. They would happen in the middle of class, while I was teaching. They would happen in the middle of the night as I tore the sheets off and tried to find pockets of cool air. My wife sometimes experienced sympathy hot flashes, drenched in sweat beside me.

Other than that, the onset of menopause or perimenopause, who can know, was fairly unremarkable. My hair thinned a bit, but because I have a thick head of hair it wasn't alarming. I didn't feel like my hormone levels were changing. I felt mostly like myself. There was some sadness because the likelihood of having a child—the old-fashioned way, with a donor and my wife wielding a turkey baster—had narrowed to a tiny sliver, but there were other options. It would be fine, no matter what. I had always known that while I would enjoy being a parent, I wouldn't feel like I lived less of a life if I wasn't one.

Menopause is, technically, a year after your last period so I don't know if I am in menopause. I'm hovering in yet another stasis, wondering if a significant part of my life is over.

———

For years, I've been dealing with writer's block though that is far too mild a term to describe it. One day, I was writing with ease, looking forward to getting back to the page each day, and the next, it was all gone. I would stare at an open Word file, the cursor slowly blinking, my fingers hovering above the keys as I willed them to make something out of nothing.

What had once been joyful instantly became misery. It was a breathtaking shock. I have always loved writing and I have always wanted to be a writer. Writing and reading have been the constants in my life so to lose them unmoored me completely. And because I was still publishing work, no one understood or believed me when I expressed how severely blocked I was, creatively. Technically, yes, I was writing but it wasn't my best. It came in fits and spurts. I hated having to share work with anyone, and doubted every word I wrote, every idea I tried to develop. My writing was stilted, flat, drab. It stunned me, really, that I was capable of producing such inadequate, lifeless prose. The longer it went on, the harder it became to write. I'm stubborn, so I kept at it, but it was always squeezing absolutely nothing from obdurate stone. I felt utterly depleted and embarrassed.

I stopped trusting my judgment, my intelligence, my voice. I lost all faith in myself as a writer. I started making alternative plans for the future, one where I could no longer credibly identify as a writer. It was grim but I so deeply believed I could no longer write that I needed to find a different way forward. On a more practical note, I needed to be able to pay my mortgage and student loans and meet my other financial obligations. At first this was all very annoying, and then it was sad, and then it was terrifying as panic set in. Deadlines came and went for days, weeks, months, and in some cases several years. The patience of my editors frayed to almost nothing and I understood. My patience with myself was similarly frayed. I felt so much shame, I thought I might drown in it.

So much of who I am is entwined with writing. I'm not talking about the public face of the work—the publications, the tours and events, the accolades. I can live without that. My original dream of being a writer was simple because I didn't know what to dream beyond wanting to write good books and maybe have them published. All I needed was to be able to hold onto that dream, but as these fallow years stretched on, I tried to accept that I might lose even that. Almost every night, I stared at the ceiling asking myself, "Who am I if I am not a writer?" It was a question I could not answer then or now.

And then, one day I was talking with a friend over dinner. We were on a double date with our spouses, a warm Los Angeles evening, sitting outside. The din of a busy restaurant surrounded us. We had nice cocktails. Great music was playing. My friend was talking about how the worst part of menopause was the brain fog. It affected almost everything she did on a daily basis; it was only with time and various treatments that the fog started to clear. It felt like a lightning bolt struck our table. I immediately peppered my friend with questions because I did not know brain fog could be a symptom of menopause. When I got home, I immediately started searching for more information and learned that many, many women deal with losing focus and becoming easily distracted and having no ability to concentrate and forgetting the very things we know for sure. Finally, I found a lifeline, the idea that maybe my overwhelming writer's block was not a personal failing rendering me beyond redemption, that maybe, the source of what ailed me was, at least in part, beyond my control and would not last forever.

⁓

It is a bitter thing, to have spent most of your life in a body you've been told you are supposed to hate, a body that is considered a placeholder for the real, more appropriate body you're meant to live in. You keep waiting for your real life to begin on that magical day when you finally discipline your body into what society prefers it to be. But sometimes, you get lucky. You stop waiting and start living. As I've tumbled into menopause, I'm supposed to believe my womanhood is ending but instead, I have been handed a new beginning.

Nearly six years ago, a woman named Debbie persisted in pursuing me until I finally accepted her invitation to go on a proper date. We had a lovely time and then there was a second date and a third and then we were officially girlfriends. We did long distance until the pandemic began. As we hunkered down in Los Angeles, we grew even closer, thriving with so much time together, just us and, before long, our pandemic puppy Max. We got engaged and we eloped under a plastic chuppah in Encino. We go on all kinds of adventures, all around the world. We've seen the mighty glaciers in Antarctica. On the steppes of Mongolia, we had the honor of sitting with a shaman who brought forth a spirit. In Uzbekistan, we stood at the center of Registan Square, in awe of the Islamic architecture around us. At a vineyard in Tuscany, we opened the windows to our hotel room and had a small picnic with a good bottle of wine, some cheese and cured meat, and watched *Avengers: Endgame* on an iPad after a long day of touristing. And many nights, we just sit on our couch at home, watching television and working away on our laptops. It sounds like a fairy tale and, in truth, it absolutely is. There is no more waiting. When is now.

N
  o
    w
     N
      o
       w
        N
         o
          w

Another truth is that this story is only a fairy tale because I started believing that maybe, just maybe, I was worthy of living a fairy tale, in this body, exactly as I am. My forties had already been pretty good when we met but then my wife made them extraordinary. I am no longer living a life suspended. I am, simply, living. For decades, it turns out, I wasn't really yearning to be treated like a woman. I was yearning to be treated like a human being. For the first time in my life, I am experiencing unconditional kindness, genuinely reciprocated passion, truly gentle touch. It was so startling, in the early going, as to almost be uncomfortable. Sometimes, it still is but I am more than willing to tolerate the discomfort. It's not that I experienced violence at the hands of previous lovers. They were simply careless. I allowed them to be. They did not understand me as someone to be handled with care, someone worthy of being handled with care. I did not understand myself as someone to be handled with care. I do not know if I am at the beginning or the middle or the end of menopause, but "the change" has changed me, nonetheless.

THE BUNNIES, AN OWL, AND ONE COYOTE THAT COMES CLOSER TO THE HOUSE THAN ALL THE OTHERS

By Pam Houston

I have a dog named Henry, who is getting ready to die, though if he were here he would tell you he is on his own timeline and if the last six months have taught me anything it's that I should stop making predictions. He would also tell you the way humans think about time is bullshit.

Henry is a six-year-old wolfhound who weighs 150 pounds. He came to me at two years old from a woman who needed some orthopedic surgeries and worried she could no longer take care of him. Other than his great size, Henry is an easy dog to care for. He loves all creatures great and small. He is happy to greet other dogs we run into on our walks but does not insist on it. He loves attention but does not demand it. He thinks of everyone as a potential friend, even his dog toys.

Henry has mitral valve failure, which means the valve between the left atrium and the left ventricle of his heart doesn't open the way it is supposed to, or maybe doesn't close the way it is supposed to, but either way it causes the blood to back up inside the first chamber, enlarging his heart.

Six months ago, Henry showed no signs of slowing down, but I took him to the vet because sometimes, especially when lying on his side, he would do some light, rhythmic groaning. Wolfhounds are groaners, especially as they age, but this seemed like a little too much groaning. Naturally skinny, Henry had been losing weight and no matter how much we fed him seemed unable to gain. That, I understand now, is because his heart and his metabolism think he is running all the time, even when he sleeps.

Henry is in atrial fibrillation a lot of the time, and when he's not, his heart still beats arrhythmically and feels like a small rock tumbling down a hillside of other small rocks. The vet in Pagosa Springs said, "The heart can't continue like that, it's too hard on it. One of these days it will just stop." She told us that if we wanted to treat Henry with anything other than the most basic heart medicine, he would need to go to Albuquerque for an echocardiogram. I wasn't sure I wanted to take him. It was late May and over one hundred degrees there, and the only thing Henry truly dislikes is the heat. I worried, given the already bad heart, the stress of a hot, ten-hour round trip to see an unfamiliar vet might take away whatever quality time he'd have if we just left him alone.

Then my friend Tami told me her truest heart dog, Taylor, now deceased, came to her in the form of a terrible smell (the seal carcasses Taylor loved to roll in at the beach), which Tami interpreted as a sign: I ought to call her favorite animal communicator, Nikki. Tami and I have been besties long enough that a visitation from a beloved deceased animal in the form of a rotted seal smell is not the kind of sign I would dare ignore.

May is a month of travel for me, so at the time of my phone appointment with Nikki, I was in a hot car in Burlington, Vermont; Henry was home on the ranch in Colorado with my husband, Mike; and Nikki was in her office in Santa Rosa. Nikki had asked that I send a photo of Henry, but did not ask for backstory on him or me. I told her about the impending appointment and my hesitancy, and asked her to ask Henry whether he felt up for the trip. Things were quiet for a while on the line on that hot and mildly smoky Vermont morning, wildfires in Quebec raging as they were. Then I heard Nikki giggle a couple of times.

"Henry would like you to know..." she said, pausing long enough to start my heart pounding, "that there are bunnies in the barn."

I felt my face break into its first real smile since his diagnosis. There *were*, in fact, bunnies in the barn. Henry had shown them to me when I was home just two days before, baby bunnies, who he wanted very much to befriend and I'd had to explain to him that might not be the best thing for the bunnies. He'd spent a couple of hours on his side of the fence watching them hop all around the corral. I laughed and Nikki laughed and said, "Henry's really funny."

"He is," I said, and it's true. Henry delights in making his people laugh.

In the corner of my brain that was still connected to a world other than the one the three of us were currently inhabiting, I wondered how Nikki even knew I had a barn.

"And...there's an owl," she continued, "and one coyote who comes closer to the house than all the others."

"Should I worry about the coyote?" I asked her.

"Oh no," she said, "he's just excited, he thinks of him as a kind of friend."

Now I was laughing and crying. This was my boy all right.

"Did he say anything about the cardiologist?" That boring corner of my brain still trying to keep the conversation on point.

"He said he really likes the hike up on the big blue ridge. He says he misses going there."

"Tell him I do too," I said. "Tell him we can't go up there yet because there's still snow."

"He is very interested in your bracelet."

"Yes," I said, twirling it on my wrist. Under that bracelet, the one I'd gotten in Namibia so I would always remember the African sky, was his favorite place to lick.

"He wants you to know you can have that same relationship with the sky at the ranch," she said.

"As with the African sky," I clarified, starting to get the hang of this new way of talking.

"He doesn't really want to talk about his illness," she said, "he just wants to keep showing me the things he loves." She laughed again. "Henry loves a lot of things."

After another minute, she said, "I told Henry if he sees the doctor you will be waiting right outside to take him home when he is finished. And I talked to the other dog, and she said she felt okay about Henry going to Albuquerque, but she wanted to make sure she'll still get her afternoon cheese."

The other dog is Livie. Who I had not mentioned, and who, I don't need to tell you, loves her afternoon cheese. When we hung up I still wasn't sure what to do about Albuquerque and also understood that was maybe beside the point. I was sure whatever world Nikki lived in, I wanted to live there too.

The cardiologist wasn't very nice to either of us, but I hear it's a terrible time for veterinarians (everyone) so I'm going to skip over that part. What matters is he confirmed the diagnosis and prescribed the life-extending medicine called Vetmedin that apparently only specialists can prescribe.

Henry and I spent that night in Santa Fe at my chosen mother's house (Mama Dia, more on her later) so he wouldn't have ten car hours in one day. It was a rough night, neither of us sleeping, Henry's heart chugging like a train—the Vetmedin would take days to reach its full effectiveness. We took short walks in the dark desert every hour just to keep from imploding. We finally drifted off around 5 a.m. and when I woke with a start at 5:45, Henry was sitting at attention in the doorway, intently watching a covey of quail peck around Dia's backyard.

Maybe you are wondering when this turns into an essay about menopause. Or maybe you can intuit how it already is.

The first thing I will say about having made it here, to sixty-one, is that it makes me weepy with gratitude. If I had died anytime before this decade, I would have missed the specific and ecstatic feeling of basic okayness with myself, such that when a thing like my conversation with Nikki happens, I can see it for all it is. A gift from the great dog god. A spiritual awakening. Permission to let Henry go. Permission to readjust the frame of the narrative from a tragically early death, or a condition I ought to have noticed sooner, to a life perfectly fulfilled by the daily existence of bunnies in the barn. Permission to fall back into the soft pillowy surface of everything I do not know about existence, and let that mystery hold me in my grief over Henry, let it quiet that old incessant voice that tells me if I had only been one more degree of perfect, I could have kept the bad thing from happening. To understand that Henry, and his covey of quail, and Nikki, and yes, even me, are perfect creatures made of love and light.

Postmenopause, like it or not, death *is* the next big thing, the next great mystery. I can hope for two decades of mind-expanding experiences like the one Henry and Nikki are providing me, but as I watch my elders, my mentors, my idols, drop off one by one, I want my own death to feel like something other than a black hole of fear looming on the horizon. I wish to identify my bunnies in the barn equivalent, and practice understanding, as Henry does, that one day with those bunnies can stand in for all eternity. Tall order, I know. But I catch glimpses of it, enough of them to believe I can muster up some grace to combat the fear.

The March before Henry got sick, I took my chosen Mama Dia to Iceland for her seventy-eighth birthday. Dia and I chose each other about a decade ago and we have been getting into trouble together ever since. For the last five years I've been in love with Iceland the same way a teenage girl is in love with a boy band. Most days I am wearing at least two articles of clothing either bearing the name of the country itself, or the name of one of the Icelandic horse barns where I ride when I'm there. My Instagram feed is very little these days except Icelandic horse competitions and waterfalls and volcanoes. I am learning Icelandic, one painstaking Pimsleur chapter at a time, even though virtually everyone in Iceland speaks English and would probably prefer I didn't try. It took me ten years of therapy and forty years of living to understand the difference between what feels good and what feels bad (more on that later) and Iceland feels so good that I get myself there at least twice a year to ride the small powerful horses that perfectly embody the Icelandic spirit. It is possible, before my life is over, I might live there.

When I took Dia to Iceland I knew it could not be a horse trip, but I also knew I'd be resentful if I didn't book a couple of half-day rides for our first two days in Iceland at my favorite barn, about an hour out of Reykjavik. I'd get the riding out of my system while Dia soaked off her jet lag in our hotel's glorious natural hot pools.

On the second morning, Dia decided to come to the barn with me and go for a shorter, easier ride while I went off with a different guide, just the two of us, to the soft sands of the Ölfusá

River, which is an excellent place for a gallop. I got to ride Salka, my favorite horse in all the world, who is powerful, fast, bossy, and brave. Sometimes Salka and I get to fly together, and it is the closest thing to pure freedom I have ever felt. That morning we had so much fun galloping on the riverbank we continued to gallop half the way home along the gravel horse paths that parallel nearly all of the roadways in Iceland.

We were approaching an S curve and a slight uphill, really flying. Icelanders don't exactly believe in two-point position, but I am not light on a horse's back so I try to take care of any horse I ride by getting out of the saddle when we go for an extended run. I was up there in my stirrups, in a kind of no-man's-land, when Salka, for the first time in our history, shied.

Neither the guide nor I knew what caused it: a whooper swan rising off the drainage ditch; a piece of the plastic they use to wrap hay blown in on the wind; maybe just whatever thoughts run through a smart mare's brain. Salka arced sharply out to the left, onto the hard top, and I arced with her but too hard and lost my balance. For a hopeful few seconds I thought I might pull it out, but as her zig completed itself with a zag, I realized I had to kick free, and did. I don't know how fast we were going. I know Icelandics regularly reach a speed of thirty miles per hour, so let's call it somewhere around twenty-five.

Unfortunately, what hit the paved road first was my head. Fortunately, I was wearing my helmet. Fortunately, my friend Heather had said to me, nearly three years before, "If horses are going to be your midlife crisis, you need to invest in a helmet, and a really good one." I am challenged, by language's limitations, to convey exactly how loud the sound of my own head hitting the pavement was. Kind of like a small bomb exploding inside my skull. Kind of like the ring of the world's biggest bell if my head was the clapper.

I didn't realize it at the time, but I must have been knocked unconscious, at least for a few seconds, because when we got back to the barn I saw I'd peed my riding tights. I was aware of enough shoulder pain to know it had taken some of the impact, but it was hard, in the moments after, to pay attention to anything other than the echo of the big bang still ringing in my head.

The next thing I knew I was up and running to the top of the hill where Salka waited for me, head down, like the good good girl she is. I was so amazed to be alive after a noise of that volume, some part of me didn't quite believe I was. But then I had the reins in my hand, and then I was throwing myself back up into the saddle. I was calling to the guide, who was looking at me with equal parts fear and wonder, "Let's go down to the start of that straightaway and gallop that S curve again." She was new to guiding and a tiny bit afraid of me. She followed me down to the start of the run.

Not once did I think of the Raymond Carver story, *A Small Good Thing*. Not once did I think of Natasha Richardson. When I started riding Icelandics in earnest at fifty-seven years old I knew I was making a deal with the devil, but now the worst thing had happened, and here I was back in the saddle getting ready to run. We galloped the hill again, albeit in a more controlled fashion. Then we tölted most of the way home.

It was only when we got to the barn and I started to shed my layers of coats and sweaters and neck gaiters that I realized my head was bleeding. Somewhat significantly. I had soaked three neck gaiters, the backs of two sweaters, a vest, and a coat. I'd hit the ground so hard the rear strap of my helmet, the one that does all that fancy protective work, had sliced into the back of my head. My friend Anna, who manages the barn, went to a closet and got whatever they use to treat horse wounds and poured a bunch of it on the place I was bleeding.

"You sure you're okay?" she asked about a million times before we finally got out of there. I gave Salka a big kiss on the muzzle and assured her I would see her again.

Dia and I planned to drive along the coast between seaside villages for the afternoon, but once I started driving, I felt woozy enough to know I ought not be behind the wheel.

"Let's go soak in the hot springs," I said to Dia, and she agreed.

Dia has had many jobs in her lifetime and one of those is nurse. It had been a while since her license expired, but knowledge has no expiration date. She said my eyes didn't look particularly concussion-y and I decided to believe her. She said the wound on my scalp was probably between the skin and the scalp, rather than between the scalp and the brain, which also seemed like good news. We slapped a maxi pad on my head, securing it in place with my final unbloodied neck gaiter. I wish I could say it was the first time I wore a maxi pad on my head but anyone who has spent their life with horses knows I would be lying. We invited Anna over to our hotel for dinner and ate and laughed well into the night.

I posted a photo of me and Salka on Facebook, mentioning my fall and my bleeding scalp, which was seeming, as the hours went by without a brain bleed, more and more like a surface wound, blaming myself for pushing our luck after a beautiful morning of riding, expressing my gratitude Salka wasn't hurt in any way and admitting, in the standard nonlogic of people who devote themselves to horses entirely, that the fall made me feel closer to Salka than ever before. The next morning Dia and I would leave for a nine-day drive on the Ring Road that encircles the island, dodging a series of blizzards that would start behind us and stop in front of us with such impeccable timing it would feel like we were perpetually winning some kind of game show.

The reaction I found on Facebook the next morning shocked me. Not because somebody insisted I must, right that second, turn the car around and go back to Reykjavik to see a doctor, but because nearly *everybody* did. I am talking about hundreds of people. Some were stern, some were angry, some pleaded, some shamed. They brought up Natasha Richardson. They brought up their sister's husband's cousin's neighbor who didn't go to the hospital and died. A phrase that came up with almost uncanny regularity was *you must rule out*... and several things followed. A lot of people told me what to ask the doctor to look for.

When I didn't respond with a follow-up post saying I was in an ambulance on my way back to Reykjavik, they began to direct message me. They looked up my UC Davis email and wrote me there. They sent letters to my professional website.

They found me on Instagram and WhatsApp. I understand that many of these people, possibly all of them, were showing genuine concern for me, even though, for the most part, they are people I do not actually know, as they say, IRL. It was the first time I had ever made a decision and something just shy of a thousand people reached out to tell me I had made a bad one. It invited some contemplation on my part.

The thing is, I haven't had great luck lately when I try to see a doctor of Western medicine. Mostly I can't get in, or if I can it is someone who got their degree last Tuesday, and then if I try, in the very few minutes I am given, to tell them what is actually happening in my own body—which I ought to be a qualified witness to, if not an actual expert in—they invariably act impatient, insulted, or bored. Thus we arrive at another definition of menopause: a time of life when women have accumulated enough hubris to believe they know more about what's going on inside their body than anybody else. My acupuncturist, who took the time to save my life when I was dying from long COVID, after a series of Western doctors told me, basically, that I was hysterical in the Charlotte Perkins Gillman sense, believes I know more about my body than she does. We treat Western doctors like gods in the United States even though they are never in the room with us long enough to notice our eye color let alone talk to us for real. I've long been suspicious of Western medicine's penchant for spot treatments, for cutting out and poisoning, rather than considering the body as an ecosystem, capable of healing itself. I've long worried whether Western medicine's early-detection-of-everything machines don't lead to unnecessary and expensive surgeries. I say this knowing I could need and enlist the help of Western medicine tomorrow. I say this as Henry lives on thanks to his fancy cardiologist-prescribed pills.

If I had really thought a doctor in Reykjavik, whom I would have trusted far more than a doctor in the United States (see any statistic in any recent decade comparing the health outcomes in the United States with those of its "peer" nations), could rule out my death, even in the short term, could guarantee that I would have another decade or two to love what is left of the wild and beautiful earth and some of its human and animal inhabitants, I might have driven back the hour in the wrong direction to see them. But if there is one illusion the one-two punch of long COVID and the every-man-for-himself, gun-toting hellscape imagined by our forty-fifth president (and embraced by so many of my neighbors) relieved me of, it is the one where I live forever. Not one of us can rule out our own death. We are all absolutely going to do it.

At seventy-eight, Dia has an even more laissez-faire attitude about death than I do. We had ten more days of radical fun ahead in Iceland, and the Ring Road was calling. If I had the brain bleed everyone on Facebook predicted for me and we careened off a slippery cliff into the Arctic Sea, it might save us from a much more prolonged and painful death that could be right around the corner, or years of nursing home hell. This had been among the things that returned me, postmenopause, to horses. What better moment to cash in your final paycheck, than just after re-realizing the possibility of flight.

The next night of our trip, from my tiny bunk on a farm stay on the southeasternmost tip of Iceland, I thanked the Facebook ladies for their concern, assured them Dia was feeding me arnica tablets at regular intervals, and that we were getting into healing hot water every chance we got. I couldn't turn my head more than an inch or two in either direction and I did have a niggling worry I had cracked a vertebrae in my neck, but paralysis never ensued. I felt a little better each morning, and even in the forty-mph winds and occasional whiteouts, I kept our little Dacia Duster on the highway. Any one of a million moments of pure fun during those ten days would have made a beautiful ending, but the universe conspired to get us back home.

At the Reykjavik airport, waiting for our flight, I texted with my friend Kaveh Akbar about the trip, and the fall, and he reminded me of the way addicts and children of addicts regularly walk around in agony for days or weeks because they have learned to ignore pain along with every other health-related message their body sends them. Kaveh himself once spent days in his apartment with a broken pelvis, slithering around like a snake, before a friend convinced him to go to the hospital. Dia has forty-two years of sobriety and my parents took their alcoholism all the way to their graves, so we come by our membership to this club authentically.

I told Kaveh about a time at the ranch, decades ago, when I was getting ready to host one of the weeklong workshops that back in those days made it so I could pay my mortgage. A friend named Kim was helping me with the cooking and pre-workshop cleanup. I had bought, at the Whole Foods, a key lime cheesecake, which I was planning to serve a few hours later when the students arrived. Kim and I finished our chore list and decided to take the dogs on a pasture walk. My oldest dog at the time, Dante, couldn't do the walks on hot days anymore so we left him behind.

When we returned from our walk, the box top on the key lime cheesecake had been flipped open, and Dante, tall in the way of Irish wolfhounds, had licked all the vanilla icing off the top of the cheesecake, leaving the limey rest of it almost perfectly intact. Kim's history with her alcoholic parents was at least as brutal as mine, which explains why we exchanged not so much as a word before we both sprung into action.

Kim got a bowl out of the cabinet and started mixing up butter and confectioner's sugar. I got a knife from the drawer and began doing my best to re-level the cake. Kim cut a lime into extra-thin slices to replace the decorations that had sat on top of the former layer of vanilla frosting. The writers arrived and when the first forkful of cake hit my mouth I looked for and found Kim's eyes across the room. The cake was delicious, lime and vanilla, tinged with the unmistakable flavor of dog saliva. We scanned the room but nobody else stopped smiling or eating. The workshop was off to a good start.

What makes this my favorite personal child-of-alcoholics story is that there was not one moment when either Kim or I considered, silently or aloud, the possibility we ought to throw out that cake. No, we just galloped that horse right back up the S curve. We slapped a maxi pad on our heads and drove five hundred kilometers in the opposite direction of civilization.

"It would have taken out a whole day of the trip!" Dia says now, a little defensively. "Maybe more!" which she follows with, "You know if I had thought you were really in trouble I would have insisted we go back to Reykjavik."

But I don't know that. Not exactly. And that is one of the reasons Dia is my chosen mama forever. We co-conspired perfectly not to ruin our trip to Iceland, and for whatever reason we got away with it. And even if the Facebook ladies were right about this one—and I can admit they probably were—objectivity and reason lose whatever shine they had here in these later decades, get replaced, maybe, with something closer to multiplicity, with letting intuition rule the day whenever possible, and fun and joy, and maybe even recklessness, with having, as the kids say, fewer and fewer fucks to give.

In high summer, months after Iceland and in a groove where it seemed Henry's medicine was really helping, I got an email from Dr. Andrew Loiseaux, my one true therapist. Drew was the one who got down and dirty with me around the time of my Saturn return and for a couple of decades after. The one who opened the trunk full of PTSD I'd been hauling around, locked, since childhood, the one who introduced me to EMDR, who taught me the difference between what felt good and what felt bad. The one who convinced me feelings wouldn't kill me.

His name means bird, in French, so it's no coincidence he schooled me in the mechanics of flight in my thirties and forties, helping me to say yes when the opportunity came in the form of Salka at sixty-one. It is hard to imagine who I would be now, *if* I would be now, without his brilliance and love and good care.

In addition to a personal note and a request to see me in September when he would return from his farm in Ecuador to Denver, the email contained two attachments, a letter he had sent to friends a year ago April when he was first diagnosed with bulbar ALS, and a letter from this April, describing the deterioration of his physical health over the intervening year, his frustration with and acceptance of all the ways ALS was diminishing his life.

There are probably only a handful of good ways to die, but bulbar ALS might be the absolute worst. The daily diminishments in motion, strength, speech, in the ability to eat, the fear of drowning in your own saliva, and all the while, your brain completely intact, firing like always, your body not reacting as it should.

I hadn't communicated with Drew in a long time. Not voice to voice, not even by email. But because he took up permanent residence in my head all those years ago, it feels as though I talk to him daily. He helps me make every decision. He stands behind me, quietly supportive when I have to speak up for myself, when I am being undervalued or mistreated. He talks me down from the ledge whenever I am scared or in despair.

For something close to a decade, I'd been picturing Drew in Peru, growing bananas, communing with lemurs and beautiful birds. I'd been wrong about which country he was in, and wrong about my belief that by virtue of his goodness he might live forever. Now he was coming back to take Colorado up on its offer of assisted suicide when his quality of life slipped below a certain level. The email suggested a window of weeks we might meet.

I definitely wanted to see him. Also, I was afraid.

When I had first started seeing Drew in my thirties, my friend Betsy and I figured out her kids were in school with his kids and when we were trying to make sure we had the same Drew I said, "Well, he's really tall, at least six foot three or six foot four"

"Oh," Betsy said, "then that isn't the same person."

The next time I was in Drew's office I measured us against one another. He was taller than me, but not by much, five foot nine," maybe in the slight lift of his running shoes. Which just goes to show you the problem with objectivity. To me Drew was a giant, and an immortal one at that.

I arrived at his house at 8 a.m. on a Sunday morning. I'd never been to his house because I was his patient, not his friend. The second I arrived I realized what a colossal mistake it would have been to let my fear keep me from coming. I don't think that was ever a real possibility. I would do literally anything to show him my gratitude. But now I saw how valuable the visit was going to be to me.

Drew was still in there, every bit of him, regardless of weakened arms, slurred speech, thirty fewer pounds on an already thin frame, every ounce of the man who held space for me to become a whole person resided there, behind his eyes. I forced myself not to cry, ironic, since he had been the one who taught me how. I was afraid he'd think I was crying at his physical diminishment, when really it was the sheer joy of seeing him that brought tears to my eyes.

Back when, in our work together, a typical session would go like this:

Drew would say, "How did that make you feel when he told you he was spending the weekend with his ex?"

And I would say, "Well, I think it would be mature of me to feel good about their friendship."

And he would say, "How did that make you feel when your mother called your roommate and tried to convince her to take you to Weight Watchers?"

And I would say, "Well, I think my mother and I have different value systems around body image."

And he would say, "How did it make you feel when your mother didn't stop your father from dragging your eight-year-old self into the shower with him, or going into your room at night?"

And I would say, "I think my mother was very breakable, and there was a silent agreement between us that we would use my body to protect her from her pain."

And he would say, "How did it make you feel when your short story got picked for Best American Short Stories of the Century?"

And I would say, "Well, I think I was lucky it was John Updike picking because I know he has a soft spot for voice."

What we both understood, of course, is I didn't know how I felt about anything.

Somehow, I was writing books that moved people, I was

teaching classes that helped others access their deepest selves, so there had to have been some kind of feeling in there. But I could not begin a sentence with the words "I feel" to save my life. The world came at me, as if I were one of those big padded contraptions football players slam into over and over. Good things, bad things, all things, hit me head-on, and I did my best just to keep my feet.

Teaching for a week at the Community of Writers conference at what is now called Palisades Tahoe decades ago, I was slated to give a reading with the great Gary Snyder on the top of the mountain. Also at the top of the mountain was a platformed bungee jump, and the conference organizers had the idea that it would be really cool if I took the leap. This was long before Instagram, of course, but in the same spirit. Community of Writers would put a photo of me jumping on next year's conference program. I was a river guide at the time and generally outdoorsy, so they figured bungee jumping was a natural extension of that.

I no more wanted to bungee jump than carve out my spleen with a rusted spoon. I had zero interest in man-made thrill-seeking contraptions, thought them, in fact, obscene, and I had little interest in being the cover of next year's brochure. But I agreed to bungee jump because even then, well into my thirties, I believed if somebody said it, I had to do it. That once a thing existed out in the air it had to be satisfied. This belief led me, in my young life, to dive off bridges into shark-infested waters, to jump off couloirs tetchy for avalanche, to get on horse after horse that had been deemed unrideable. I was taken for a badass but I was not a badass. I was a young woman, who, thanks to her father, believed my body would always be a vehicle for the satisfaction of somebody else's idea.

That evening near Tahoe, the writers rode the gondola to the top of the mountain, some of them so afraid of heights we had to make a circular wall around them with ourselves. We disembarked and clustered near the giant mats underneath the bungee. Alone, I climbed the however many flights of stairs to the platform. I already had the giant rubber bands affixed to my ankles when it hit me with true clarity how much I did not want to jump.

The terror I felt on the platform might have been the first moment of pure feeling since before memory, since before my father taught me what my body was for. The ski bro running the jump shamed me in all the predictable ways as he unwrapped the rubber bands from my ankles. The third time in two minutes he told me there were no refunds I said I would give him a hundred dollars to shut the fuck up.

In the mountaintop lodge, where I warmed up the crowd for Gary Snyder, I opened with a sincere, nearly tearful apology. "I'm sorry," I said, "I know I let you all down. There is nothing to say about it except I was terrified."

After the reading Gary came up to me and said, "Pam, you know we're all secretly glad you didn't jump." It took another decade to realize he was being truthful as well as kind.

Drew taught me a whole new language. Pleasure and pain, fear and joy, happiness, as well as terror, and the bodily sensations that assisted in their identification. I didn't always get the answer right, but I increasingly knew I was feeling something. That lift under my breastbone when the feeling is joy, the feeling I still get, every single time my plane touches down in Iceland. With fear, the first tell is that I cease making eye contact. I know this is all entirely obvious. It just wasn't obvious to me.

At Drew's house, his wife did a lot of the talking for him because his vocal cords could not keep up with his brain. When he did talk I mostly understood him. When I didn't understand him, I asked him to repeat. I pledged not to fake anything in front of this man who taught me to stop faking everything. If I had cried at the door, I realized, it would have been perfectly okay. I stayed for nearly two hours. We talked about courage and rage and acceptance. We talked about all the books we had read lately and loved. He said when he is lost in a truly engaging novel is the only time he forgets he has ALS, so I vowed to send him all my recent favorites. We talked about assisted suicide as the last true mercy a person can show himself. He was thinking he would choose that path sometime after the holidays. I wanted to stay forever to be near the spark of his eyes, the wisdom that so clearly lived there, but he was tired and I had a long ride back to the ranch and Henry.

"You taught so many of us how to live," I told him. "Now you are going to teach us how to die."

A week after I visited Drew, Mike and I took Henry on a road trip because we felt his care was too much responsibility to leave with a ranch sitter, and because it seemed like Livie might be going into heat, which would provide way too much excitement, and because we'd been planning the trip for a long time. His presence changed everything about our itinerary, where we stayed, what we did with our hours, the very definition of a good day. Instead of camping out, we stayed in a stationary Airstream near Escalante, Utah. Instead of long hikes or backpacks we took short walks and looked for a stream to sit beside. A lot of our time was spent convincing Henry to eat the bison burger and sockeye salmon that now comprises his diet. Keeping a 150-pound dog who will only take small bites of food on three thousand calories a day takes up a lot of time, but beautifully.

One morning, in the middle of that week together, we thought Henry might be dying. He had a lot of fluid built up in his chest and abdomen and could not cough it up. We drove him to a stream—he has always loved a stream—and told him it was okay, that we knew how tired his heart must be, that he could go ahead and die and we would find ways to be okay without him.

Henry stood in the stream for about an hour, and it was the first hour of this entire journey it seemed he was truly suffering. His heartbeat causes discomfort, certainly, and sometimes a little fear, but I hadn't thought he'd been in pain, exactly, until that moment. After a while he came over and put his forehead hard against mine and looked right into my eyes for more than a minute.

"It's okay," I said again, "thank you for loving us. We'll be okay if you have to go."

He took one giant belly breath, climbed up on the sandy bank, curled himself into a ball and went to sleep for two hours. He woke up refreshed, wagging and ready to get in the car.

With much of the day still ahead of us, we drove over to Bryce Canyon, where he got out at every overlook and greeted people like some latter-day Jesus after the resurrection. Every single passenger on a bus full of Taiwanese tourists took photos with him, one at a time. He licked the faces of babies and children, wagged for all the ladies in spandex and Lycra, let a young man who had grown up with wolfhounds sniff behind his ears. Henry had always had a goofy aspect; now his illness had turned him into some sort of oracle. We started to feel as though we were accompanying the Dalai Lama on his farewell tour.

I know Mike and I will remember that week as one of the best we ever spent together, in love as we were with Henry and each other and the mind-bending landscapes of the Escalante plateau. The natural world is never more beautiful than when someone you love is about to leave it. Mike and Henry and I saw that beauty together, and the care we gave Henry created another new intimacy among us, which must be one of the great mercies inside anticipatory grief.

Then Mike flew back East to see his family and I started the teaching quarter at Davis with Henry in tow. There Henry got to see many of his old friends and make some new ones. It was still hot, so my friend Liz let us use her empty house in Truckee on the long weekends. We took slow walks through the peak of fall colors, took swims in Donner Lake, lingered next to many a stream. I was reminded that when I prioritize a dog's wishes, my life improves immeasurably. His failing body reminded me I have one too, and stepping away from the computer every hour or so for a micro walk does us both a lot of good. Our nights in Truckee with lots of pee outings (he also takes a diuretic) reminded me that every single hour of the day and night is beautiful, and that paying attention to the natural world with all of my senses, as he does, is the key to a rich and meaningful life.

In mid-October I drove Henry back to the ranch, and on the way he had a heart attack. We stopped to stay the night with my friend Eliza, and Henry was feeling good enough the next morning to chase a couple of horses, two gentled mustang mares. One second he was galloping after them, respectfully, on his side of the fence, and the next second he had keeled over. I ran to him, put my hand on the patch of hair that was still short from the echocardiogram, and there was no heartbeat whatsoever. His eyes stared straight ahead, glassy and blank. "I love you, Henry," I said, into the silence the stillness in his chest was making out of the morning.

Then, under my hand, like an ancient truck starting on a ten-degree morning, that poor old heart kicked up and rumbled back to life.

We were still a ten-hour drive from the ranch when it happened. I didn't know if he would make it home, but I wanted him to. I wanted him to be able to see Livie and Mike, to smell the smells, to check in with his bunnies (now rabbits) and all the other wild creatures. I wanted him to be able to lie on the porch couch and keep track of the horse and the donkey, the sheep and the chickens, to flow back into the flow of the ranch, even if only for a couple days. I drove too fast and held my breath during every pee break, cursed the construction delays and sang *You Are My Sunshine* to him over and over because Eliza said my singing would keep him alive and that was the only song my adrenaline exhausted brain could think of. We made it and Henry settled in almost immediately right next to the corral fence where he can best keep track of all his friends.

Now it is November, and Henry has had weeks of good ranch time, settling back into frosty mornings, first snow on the mountains, smells of the elk and the mule deer and the barnyard, good sandy ranch dirt beneath his paws, evenings by the fire, or out on his porch couch, under the newly rising winter stars.

I'm in California, teaching, so grateful for the month we had together, not quite daring to hope he will make it to Thanksgiving, when my schedule will allow me to see him again. Last week Henry had another heart attack, this time at the sight of his most beloved Fed Ex lady, who brings his medicine every two weeks, along with a cookie in her pocket. Once again, his determined heart sputtered back from the dead.

Henry doesn't measure time in days or weeks or medicine deliveries or semester breaks, but by the departure of the osprey and the first snow up on the La Garita Mountains. Tami says his staying this long means he has something to teach me, and I am trying, with every bit of my heart, to learn.

When I was preparing to write this essay, the first words I put on paper were, *menopause means coming to terms with myself.* I wasn't sure exactly what I meant by that.

For all my life, every time I've had a thought about anything, the thought that came right on its heels in a slightly different voice (an amalgamation of my parents and all the other people I have proved too much for over the years) was one that revealed all the ways my original thought was wrong. Not only wrong, but somehow lethal, a thought so odious it could lead, if extended far enough forward, to my own demise, or even the demise of others. What this voice says about Henry, for example, is that if I make one single mistake, in ordering his meds, or taking him on too long a walk, or not intercepting the Fed Ex lady at the bottom of the driveway, or even just by going back to California to do my job, I will be responsible for killing him.

But Henry is on his own trajectory, and I can't keep him from dying any more than my perfect behavior kept my father from hurting me. I can't keep him safe from all the wild mustangs and the treat-bearing Fed Ex ladies, or his beloved sister Livie whose butt smells so good, and if it is Henry's excitement over the smell of Livie's butt that causes his heart to stop in a fit of ecstasy, who am I to say that isn't the best possible way to die.

I have always believed there is no limit to what I can learn from animals. If I can surrender myself to the love of the bunnies, the owl, the one coyote that comes closer to the house than all the others—a thing I have watched Henry do again and again with no effort—I might become a better writer. I would certainly become a better human being. Also, there is a way Henry and I can be together when he's in Colorado and I'm in California or a hot car in Vermont, and this possibility of togetherness can go on in some aspect, even after he dies, even after Drew dies, or Dia does, or I do. Because by the time menopause rolls around we better have come to understand we are stardust, we are energy, changeable in form; and also that time is what we make of it, not to mention reality, not to mention love, which is probably all there actually is anyway. So I will wake up this morning and send kisses to Henry across the stratosphere and ask him which of his friends he saw this morning. And he will remind me that that tired old punishing voice is only coming from inside the house now, and once I fully grasp that, I'll have the power to set it free.

TRANSMOGRIFY

By Lidia Yuknavitch

I want to tell you a story shaped like a fairy tale, but the world of the story is my body. I want to show you how I have used the practice of storytelling, that is, reading stories and writing stories, even shape-shifting through each act of storytelling, to navigate menopause. I believe in narrative medicine. Anyone anywhere can tap into the power of storytelling. This book is in part a collection that illuminates how multiplying our very different stories, letting them fan out, tendril, cross one another, makes a story constellation one might take into their life in times of duress. My own addition is a kind of conjuring. Story space is a real place, though sometimes humans forget deeply enough that they recite fairy tales to children only, and they begin to lose the ability to grow tails or scales or wings or gills. Sometimes I think we have it backward. Perhaps we should let children read fairy tales to us. I am nothing if not a believer in carrying stories. My mother wanted to name me Cassandra.*

Shocking to almost no one who knows me, my favorite fairy tale is about a mermaid. Not the Disney mermaid, though she is wonderful in her various incarnations. Not the Hans Christian Andersen mermaid, though that story does of course interest me. The story that best holds my heart is Lithuanian. Some of my blood comes from a Baltic place. The Lithuanian fairy tale may predate Hans Christian Andersen. Supposedly, the tale was first recorded around 1842, in the writings of Liudvikas Adomas Jucevičius.

That last name is my paternal family's last name as well. I have no idea if the connection is just sort of trippy or more. I'm not sure I care. It is enough that we find secular synchronicities in the world that give us moments of awe—for me that is sacred—or magical—enough.†

For me, the figure of the undine, the partly human water creature, is one that helps me to remember we humans, like all living things, are always undergoing transmogrify. We are always participating in the process of moving from one form to another. We don't always slow down enough to think about those changes as a story worth meditating on. Or we find fault

---

* My father wanted to name me Eve. That difference is very telling, but not part of this story.
† On the topic of fairy tales and synchronicity, read pretty much anything by Jungian Marie-Louise Von Franz.

with the changes that come. We are often bombarded with stories from our culture that capture us inside some trap of too fat, too thin, too old, too young, not beautiful enough. Fairy tales are filled with all kinds of transmogrifies that remind us we are always and forever shape-shifting.

In many Baltic fairy tales and folktales, Jūratė is known as the mermaid goddess of the sea. In some versions she is simply an undine, one of my favorite words of all time. My grandmother— my father's mother—told me a story about the undine Jūratė. Jūratė lived in a palace made from amber, the national gemstone of Lithuania. The palace was underneath the Baltic Sea. The story goes that she fell in love with some kind of crafty mortal named Kastytis. In most versions he is a fisherman. He was definitely handsome or at least mesmerizing to Jūratė... I'm guessing like my first husband. And my second husband. And my third. Maybe he was just very good at and passionate about what he was doing. That form of attraction happens to me a lot. I see someone who is very good at what they are doing, and I am hypnotized. Drawn to them in ways I almost cannot control. Jūratė and Kastytis become lovers, and she takes him underwater to the amber palace, but this makes Perkūnas the Thunder God angry (shocking, huh), so Perkūnas smashes the palace into tiny pieces of amber, killing Kastytis. From that moment on, when Jūratė experiences her own grief and loss, her tears come out as little pieces of amber.

My earliest memories of mermaids come from me watching my mother get dressed in the bathroom when I was young.

Her disability, having been born with one leg six inches shorter than the other, put her through several bone surgeries around puberty. That alone marked her for life, slipped her—and me—into a story unlike anyone else. The long pearly scar running up the side of her leg made me think of fish scales. I was already competing as a swimmer by the age of six, so water associations were very important to me. The origin story of me as a competitive swimmer is not bound to athleticism. I believed I could breathe underwater from the moment I could talk. I would jump into any water we encountered as a family—rivers, lakes, pools, the neighbor's koi pond, and of course, the ocean. That's why they gave me swimming lessons at four years old, and that is the story of how I became a lifelong swimmer. To keep me from drowning. Or swimming home. My early experiences staring at my mother's leg shaped my imagination.

Every important event in my life has some connection to water. My daughter's ashes are buried in the Pacific Ocean. My father drowned off the coast of Florida. My mother's menopause started the day I got married for the first time, on a beach in Corpus Christi, her last blast of blood staining her white sundress in the ass. She spoke at the wedding while bleeding. I stared out at the water. I think I saw an Atlantic bottlenose dolphin, but I can't be sure. I am sure a story got born in me that day, my mother's last blood, the power of water, a dolphin, a baby secretly swimming inside me who would not live. If I could swim back and get my mother and daughter and give their lives back to them, I would.

The world's fairy tales and folktales open their own imagination portals. Another way to say that is that fairy tales and folktales time travel. They stitch themselves back and forth in time and space like star constellations, culture by culture. Underwater mermaid figures have swum across the entire globe. The Syrian goddess Atargatis, whom the gods transformed into a half-fish. In Chinese mythology there are Lingyu, who have fishtails but also feet, and Diren, who have mermaid tails. Scotland has the Ceasg or maid of the wave, Greece has that wonderful mythological creature part bird and part fish known as the Siren, and Russia has Rusalki. There is a history of mermaids in Africa known as Mami Wata. The Maliseet tribes have stories of Lampeqinuwok, or water sprites, and the Passamaquody have stories of half-fish half-humans as well, including the story of Ne Hwas, which is really about two sisters who turned into mermaids. The Paiute, Salish, Washoe, and Shoshone have a legend about Paakniwat, water babies. Japanese Ningyo have the power to cry pearls, some are fortune tellers, and they look absolutely nothing like Western images of mermaids. They might deliver good or terrible news.

Thinking about stories of mermaids releases me from the tyranny of chronology and the pathos of the personal. I've never understood aging as something different than the rest of an embodied, lived life. I mean I do understand that we go through lifelong changes in being, but I don't think of "aging" as the story I've been told about it. I am particularly baffled by the "aging woman" story. The crone archetype is interesting to me as a story, but only a little. Older women are the most sexually attractive beings on the planet to me and have been since forever. I'm not attached to the biological essentialism of a woman's body. I don't even subscribe to genders. I don't think of babies as the beginning of a life, I don't think of old as the end of a life, not in any linear way. I know how I came to this way of thinking outside the lines. I've held a dead infant in my arms too long. My daughter, whose birth and death happened simultaneously, rearranged my DNA. All of time contracted. Then expanded. She was born in and died in amniotic waters. She spilled from my body perfectly but dead. All the stories I have inherited about life and death as happening in any linear way dissolved in that moment. Forever. Mythic.

Partly how I survived the loss of my daughter is to endlessly story her in my writing. She is a creature who appears as an infant, a girl, a woman, a female who can breathe underwater, a whale, a narwhal, a seal, a mermaid, an aquanaut. Healing through storytelling has liberated me from grief and loss many times.

I've run across many theories over the years about why mythological creatures who can live underwater inhabit so many global folktales and fairy tales. Water is a profoundly transformational element, so that likely has something to do with it. Human babies begin their lives in water, and humanity began its life through water. My heart says the attraction to water creatures inside storytelling space may also reflect the human desire to return to some origin and simultaneously swim away from one's beginnings, which is certainly an impossibility in our land lives, but easily accomplished in fairy tale space.

Partly I have navigated the experience of my own aging, and menopause specifically, by aggressively searching for stories, an effort that has, let's be honest, been my go-to strategy about navigating pretty much anything in life. Honestly, I'm not sure I have any other life skills. Writing stories is what I have to give. In particular, I wanted stories about anything but aging human women. Don't get me wrong. I love human females. Particularly women who are older than I am. Maybe more than some of you seem to be aware of. But when I make myself the center of the story as an aging human, a little internal light starts flashing, warning me that humans are not the only creatures to move through metamorphoses as they age. This is a lesson I am learning as one who is aging myself. I have to make an effort to remember that we are one species among legions of other species and organisms on the planet, and when I do make the effort, everything is better.

In my quest to find helpful stories about menopause in the nonhuman world, I kept running into the importance of storytelling. Storytelling is a potent bridge to the world and to each other. Stories move us. Fictional stories, scientific stories, personal stories, spiritual stories, historical stories, cultural stories, all of which shift with time. Story space is where human knowledge and experiences cross and make constellations. When a storyteller begins to change the shape of the story, change is afoot. Think of Greta Thunberg—not as a savior, which is a different kind of story, but as someone willing to risk moving the narrative. Now think of Jane Goodall. Their age gap doesn't matter to me. The stories they share move ideas around.

I remember the first time I read *Women Who Run with the Wolves: Myths and Stories of the Wild Woman Archetype* by psychoanalyst Clarissa Pinkola Estés. Her storytelling as well as her navigational efforts through other stories in the world profoundly released me, and reminded me that the cycles of life we move through and the stories we share make a deep difference in how we feel about living our lives. Clarissa too found solace in the world's fairy tales, and in particular stories about animals. Fairy tales are filled with signs and guides, and they never move through logic. They move through magic and intuition. I identify mightily with her call to look for doors by way of your own experiences and your intuition: "If you have a deep scar, that is a door; if you have an old, old story, that is a door. If you love the sky and the water so much that you almost cannot bear it, that is a door." Another book that blew my doors open more recently was Alexis Pauline Gumbs's incredible *Undrowned: Black Feminist Lessons from Marine Mammals*. In brief lyric movements she moves through water and language by way of marine mammals. She points to the ways in which both storytelling and the power of metaphor are portals to important social justice work with each other as well as internally for the individual. Her call is to "see what happens when I rethink and refeel my own relations, possibilities, and practices inspired by the relations, possibilities and practices of advanced marine mammal life."*

Though I first met her on the pages of her book *How Animals Grieve*, Barbara J. King has become someone whose work I turn to often now as I move through this part of my life. She has also become a friend. I asked her about her lifework in anthropology and her research into animals and menopause. She shared with me ideas about the importance of "biocultural"† ways of thinking about animal behaviors. We talked about recent research on chimps and menopause, of course. I have a lifelong love affair with chimps that got born sometime around puberty in my life, the day I first read Jane Goodall's book *My Life with Chimpanzees*. Barbara sent me the most recent research articles on chimps and menopause, which were, in a word, thrilling.‡

Barbara and I also had a brief exchange on the wonder of female cetaceans, particularly short-finned pilot whales, killer whales, narwhals, and beluga whales. Her thoughts brought me back again to storytelling:

---

* Alexis Pauline Gumbs, *Undrowned: Black Feminist Lessons from Marine Mammals* (2020).

† Biocultural analyses seek explicitly to overcome the limitations of turning biology and culture into a binary.

‡ Kasha Patel, "We Now Know Female Chimps Go Through Menopause. Here's Why That's a Big Deal," *Washington Post*, October 26, 2023, https://www.washingtonpost.com/climate-environment/2023/10/26/female-chimpanzees-menopause-discovery/.

What joy to contemplate how the long lives of these female cetaceans brings them—embedded as they are in cultures of knowing and loving and learning and grieving—new opportunities as they age. Over their lives, they flourish in cultural and individual ways of being daughters, mothers, grandmothers, as both themselves and also integral parts of their groups. I have come to think in terms of animals' narrative arcs, comprehensively—so many other-than-human animals create their own stories... to be a menopausal mammal is to do this in ways that may bring new worlds into being!

Narrative arcs are my jam, particularly when those arcs make shapes we might find in the natural world, like waves or spirals or radiating circles or rhizomatic clusters. Clarissa Pinkola Estés is a post-trauma recovery specialist, psychoanalyst, and activist. Barbara J. King is an anthropologist, writer, and activist. Alexis Pauline Gumbs is a poet and activist. I am drawn to the ways their stories intersect.

Sometimes I think the hard line between science and storytelling limits our imaginations. Just look up at the night sky. Witness a constellation. Ask yourself what the science is. Then ask yourself what the story is. The night sky, like the ocean, and really, the entire planet, is a place where science and story are always locked in a kiss. As Rebecca Solnit reminds us in *Storming the Gates of Paradise: Landscapes for Politics*, "The stars we are given. The constellations we make. That is to say, stars exist in the cosmos, but constellations are the imaginary lines we draw between them, the readings we give the sky, the stories we tell." I am *not* saying we should be attracted to fuzzy science. I respect knowledge gatherers mightily. And I thank my lucky stars that science exists. I'm just saying we all intersect at the level of story and imagination, and that place is real, and powerful, and worth amplifying.

To enter the story of how I shape-shifted I must turn away from feeling like humans are the most important beings on the planet, turn away from the story of a heteronormative biologically determined body, one whose chief value is reproductive, and turn toward stories of animals, mythological figures, and the transmogrify of fairy tales. For me, story space is a collective creativity ocean. My own transmogrify is a kind of reverse mermaid story.

First you must picture my body. I don't want to scare you by talking about how hard I am trying to grow a mermaid tail. So just imagine a tattoo—black lines forming mermaid scales running from my heel up the side of my leg past my hip up my torso all the way to my armpit. Can you see them? Yes, there was some difficulty to endure. The markings on my body took six hours. The tattooing overrode all the other woes in my life at the time, because pain that is willingly entered through ceremony is a transformational space. But the pain I endured was nothing compared to the true difficulties I have faced in my life. That's the thing about chosen rituals. They carry with them the possibility of liberation and transformation.

The tattoo marked the decade of my fifties. That decade was

the third time in my life I entered a cavernous woe cave. The first was surviving my father's abuse as a child, the second was surviving the death of my daughter. The woe that came during my fifties, the body crucibles of menopause and the heaviness of spirit, felt like some kind of spell from nowhere that landed on my body, my heart. I didn't think at the time, "go get a tattoo to ease your menopause journey, woman!" But I do believe from this distance I can say that my intuition was way ahead of me. Hopefully some of our shared stories here will give you a leg up.

Additionally, the tattoo pain was nothing like the pain my mother endured her entire life as a woman whose pain in her hip and leg ate her alive, day by day, year after year, likely contributing to her choice to enter the liquid life of a vodka. Her disability originally put her in the hospital in a body cast for almost a year during puberty, more than one surgery planted a lifelong steel plate lodged at her hip, a long pearling scar ran up the shorter leg. As I say, my tattoo was a choice. My mother was born into pain. Sometimes my tattoo talks to her scar in a language no one else understands. I mean in my imaginal world. My mother, like my daughter, is dead, but I story my way to them often. If that is not the magic of story space, I don't know what is.

The second thing you must imagine is a magical spell. During this tattoo trial, I talked out loud toward the world and I spoke internally to myself. For example, I said the word "motherfucker" so many times, the word itself began to shape-shift, exactly the same way that Gertrude Stein said it would when she lectured on repetition and rearrangements of meaning. I encourage you to look that up in *Lectures in*

America. The word began to change. There was of course the profane meaning, a response to pain. But the more times I said "motherfucker," both out loud as well as inside my head, the more meanings emerged. Fuck you, mother. Patriarchy fucks mothers. Mothers fuck shit up. Mothers will fuck your shit up. Mothers who fuck unite. To be mothered is to be fucked. Fuck motherhood. Fuuuuuuuck, *motherhood.* The mother of all fuckers. Pretty soon the entire lexicon we call language opened up into endless motherfucker expanse, the pain of getting the tattoo transformed into pleasure, I cried and I laughed simultaneously, one of the most glorious states of being available. I may have peed. If I did, apologies to my queer tattoo artist, a writer, artist, and healer, though I feel certain he would understand. I did nearly kick him in the jaw when he was working down by my ankle. I wish my feet had gone to fin right then and there. No, I am not suggesting we all start chanting motherfucker more often, although, I can think of worse ideas. I'm asking, what magical word or story or spell might you conjure that gives you courage and hope?

The third thing you will need is a magical object for the journey of this story, especially if you are willing to travel the underworld, as I did, initially. Fairy tales always hold a kind of promise, so put that promise in your heart pocket like a talisman for travel. I suggest a small and beautiful rock that fits into the palm of your hand. Or a shell. Or a feather. An old coin or a button. I mean come on. You know how to travel fairy tales. You do. You choose the object. Remember you can speak to this object in addition to holding it and carrying it.

262 THE BIG M

And listen, you do not have to dive down into the underworld if you do not want to, however, I hope that one or two people do—I could have used a twin or a comrade or even a mechanical owl at the time. But I understand that not everyone needs to enter the underworld in order to transform. I mean what a crock. What a load of shit we've been fed concerning the crucibles we must pass through in order to earn the right to claim full humanity. The hero's journey, which counts some bodies as heroic and others as evil or nothingness, sacred scriptures that position women in impossible spaces such as immaculate conception...I mean JESUS, way to take sexuality and reproduction away from actual women's bodies and donate that power to various menfolk minions who wear long robe dresses and serve an invisible man in the sky (thanks no thanks Christianity), and all the narrative positions of witch, monster, whore, jealous queen, lowly servant...the list is long, global, and annoying. It's almost as if the space of "woman" is not counted as fully human. Anyone who steps into that space, watch your ass.

At any rate. Should you have the desire to travel through what I felt was the underworld, here is the portal.*

———————————

* In my late forties, around forty-eight, I thought I might be dying. There are some big health tremors in my genetic code, both paternal and maternal, like most people these days, I suppose. And WebMD has turned so many of us into obsessive internet moles, digging down into a doom vortex. I think you'd agree it has become fairly easy to panic when you don't feel right. Or even if you feel anything at all.

My personal Hades invaded my whole body. Headaches and nausea and abdominal pain ascended like locusts. Fatigue unlike all the other kinds of fatigue I had ever experienced overtook me at inopportune moments. I mean, the fatigue of puberty, with its hormonal juts and starts, the fatigue of motherhood, with its nut-ball matrix of impossible tasks, the fatigue of relationships and too many full-time jobs on top of each other (wife, mother, teacher, writer, colleague, friend, daughter, sister, cook, housecleaner) were already under my belt. But the fatigue that came in my late forties would find me gently resting my head on the car window at a gas station, or dropping down dramatically on the floor of my academic office, or driving to a park and collapsing underneath a tree. My body temperature went haywire as well. Heat would rise to the surface of my skin in fire bursts. Like a series of fevers from nowhere. Often in the middle of teaching a college class, or at an important dinner or event—you know, public places where I was meant to appear calm and cool or in control. I had zero control over these flushed furies. And they brought with them some kind of brain spin. I'd be in the middle of a sentence and lose the rest of the sentence, or any meaning the sentence might have originally intended. I'd be standing there open-mouthed, witless, and burning. Like a human match. Like rip-your-clothes-off hot, though thankfully, I didn't do that, at least not in the classroom. My car parked in the parking lot of the community college I taught at became more and more elusive at the end of each day.

My periods, which had been steadfastly and boringly regular for thirty years, went berserk. They came too often or not at all or with an overwhelming gush and clot that I began to refer to as the Red Sea. One night I called my husband into the bathroom to witness with me. Do you think that's normal? We stared at the red stuff in the toilet. We were both frightened. I lost the ability to sleep through the night. My nights became a staccato toss and turn punctuated by sweat and profanity. When my husband amorously reached for me in the night, or in the morning, I wanted to kill him. I may have growled.

Simultaneously, my appetites became expansive. I wanted to eat every food on the planet, drink all the wine and single malt scotch, smoke all the pot. My desire dislocated from time, space, and humans, though many humans looked humpable to me. In truth, most humans, especially other women. Trees, water, the couch, the ocean, chairs, pillows endlessly attracted me...the erotics of cooking, dancing, bathing, swimming, even reading books got me off quickly and abundantly. I developed a curious new habit of masturbating on airplanes, right there in the seat. I nearly rubbed my nub off masturbating all over the place, and the house filled with new toys and tricks, which made up for the cock-block instances.

I had a new brat sister self too. Her name was Rage. It felt to me like a creature I had locked in a small box my entire life had suddenly escaped, and she and I were in a fierce battle for the territory of my body and mind. Rage had serpents for hair. Rage had potty mouth. Rage's breasts fired rockets and her vagina had teeth. Rage was infuriated by the opinions of others. Any opinions. Rage was judgy as fuck. Rage had some issues. She erupted any time she wanted, she overtook situations like she'd been running the show forever, she was irrational, sexy in a terribly excessive way, and loud. Rage drank too much and she was packing heat. And Rage had a lover: Mood Swings, who swung to the moon and back quite violently and without warning.

But none of these strange, staggering feelings compared to what became something of an ongoing and seemingly endless nightmare for me: recurring urinary tract infections. As the walls of my uterus thinned and my estrogen dropped, I began to have a new UTI each *month*. One of which became so serious it turned into a kidney infection that nearly aced me, leaving me with a bum kidney for life. If this happens to you please know there is help, there are options. I was terrified but didn't have to be. There is help. Tell someone immediately. Tell everyone. Seek out a women's health clinic, and an acupuncturist, in addition to your primary care physician. Call in other women, dead or living. Read stories. Keep holding onto the magic rock or other object as we go deeper into story space. The objects we collect and carry with us accumulate magic, just like metaphors do. The small ceremonies and rituals we invent could very well save our lives, sharing stories being an important example.

As I moved from my forties into my early fifties, I began to disassemble. My marriage fractured. My body was at war with itself. I began to eat too many Vicodin—partly for chronic spine pain (I have scoliosis so my body changes were creating a kind of spinal crisis), partly for crippling depression, partly because like my mother, I am an addict. So the idea that I could just become liquid eased the pain some. I put on pounds. Exactly thirty-five pounds. My breasts seemed to be increasing daily, like expanding watermelons. I had some concern that if my rack got any bigger, I'd fall over frontward. I did ask a trusted friend at the time, "What if they don't stop?" And she replied, "Maybe lose weight?" She was younger than me, but not by much. Briefly I wished my own anus would just suck me up and away forever.

My teaching wavered between angry and apathetic. Sometimes I just didn't go to work. Or I'd drive to work but sit in the car drinking tiny awful bottles of Sutter Home, which came in four-packs. Sometimes I just didn't get out of bed. Sometimes my son would just sit with me while I cried about nothingness. I did not know it at the time, but I had stepped through the portal to perimenopause, which I knew exactly zero about, except what I'd read and *taught for twenty years* in Women's Studies classes. What I'm saying is, it is not true that I did not know anything. My knowledge was formidable. My copy of *Our Bodies, Ourselves* had the look of a well-worn bible. And I'd read reams of current research. But knowing a thing doesn't necessarily prepare you for living a thing. Does it.

So I think it is fair to say that I *did* know that I was at the age where radical change was afoot, but I did not want it to be true, because the stories we inherit are often monstrous, if we inherit anything at all. Blessings upon those people who have phenomenal support systems and intergenerational wisdom at their fingertips. Compassion for those of you who instead have jack shit, whatever the reasons. I suspect what devoured my own possible wisdom was

If you would prefer to enter the fairy tale without having to move through the underworld, do it. Begin again here. Instead

---

fear and loathing. Like I was eating my own heart. The fear was about aging out of something I couldn't quite put my finger on. The loathing was about not knowing where my body would end up. Or maybe both the fear and the loathing were me trying not to become my mother.

I also did not want to be the person who can't handle what is happening to me in front of other humans. Pretty sure we call that the lovely little feature ego.

Had someone wonderful thrown me a party, or better yet, since as an introvert I find parties excruciating, had someone who loved me created a glorious and previously unheard of ritual through which I might pass and be initiated into something phenomenal, you know, one in the woods or in the ocean that included perhaps a crown made from thistles, sea shells, starfish, and kelp, maybe my fear or shame would not have eaten me. Maybe all I needed was a bonfire, I don't know. Had I been better at staying connected to other humans, or better at giving myself what I know I need, I may have experienced my favorite emotion: awe. I'm saying all this out loud to remind you what you can give to yourself, what you can ask for, what you can create. What I needed was to invent rituals, ceremonies, to mark my shape-shifting. And I did give myself these things later, but I forgive myself for not knowing how to give them to myself sooner. I am hoping by sharing my underworld I can demystify it. It's just a forest. The trees are not menacing. The animals can help. I'm hoping the stories we give you will help you to move differently through your own body story. When there is pain, know that the pain is changing you. When there is fatigue, know that rest will take new forms. When there is heat, count your breaths and splash your body with cool water, when you are awake at night, tell yourself stories in your head, or write, or read, or watch bits of a series; the nights will return to you unburdened later. You are not alone, but you are going to have to conjure your own story. Reach out to all the others.

of a mermaid who falls for a clever mortal on land, I conjured a story of a person who lives on land trying to get back to water. I actually believe that in this part of my life I am making my way back to my better world. And the creatures I am falling for are not human. Seals, whales, narwhals, and always the element of water. Here is the fairy tale I am sharing with you about my own transmogrify:

Once there was a woman who fell in love with water. Oh there were handsome young men and women and ungendered creatures all around her whom she might have fallen in love with. There were children to love, parents, friends, siblings. There were beloved coworkers. There were animals and trees and gods—lots of gods of this or that. Whole epochs' worth. But nothing ever drew her love deeper than water. Not even air. It is said that she lived many years trying to find other beings and places to rest her love, to give her longing a nap, a break, but nothing worked. Inside her the longing rose in waves bigger than a body. If she lived in the forest, she was drawn to rivers. If she lived on a mountain, she was drawn to rain. If she lived in a city, she would stand too long in the shower, pitifully, or swim in chlorinated pools subjugating her desires. She wore a human smile by mimicking everyone around her. She worked hard in the world just like other workers. When she cried, she saved the tears and put them back into the ocean. She loved the people around her as best she could, but people noticed they could never attach to her, not fully. She'd just slip through their hands, or hearts. They told stories about that behind her back. She knew. She just didn't care. Her heart sang only to water. Her body belonged only to water. She felt most herself when she was alone, in water, with her eyes closed.

One night a handsome prince kissed her awake from slumber. Or maybe he was just a snappy dresser with a charismatic air. What the hell? she asked. Why would you interrupt my dream? Dreams keep me alive. She gave him a cheese sandwich and shooed him away, then went back to dreaming of water. Another night a handsome woman kissed her awake. Honestly, what is with you people kissing unconscious folk? That seems pretty creepy? She sent the handsome woman away too, with a rock. Next a weird little dwarf man visited, a drop-dead gorgeous she-witch, a centaur, an octopus (the octopus did indeed give her pause), all manner of fairy tale figures—some evil, some good, some handsome, some not, no one and nothing could capture her imagination or desire like water could. She found all the attention annoying and a little pathetic. Wasn't it obvious she was not, nor ever would be, the object of anyone else's desire? She was no object. She would not stand inside any story that positioned her thus. Ever.

And so she waited for the day or night when the sea—her real love—would call her home. Unlike most people she knew, she never, not once, doubted the sea. Each night she would visit water and hold open her arms, waiting for the embrace. She knew she would either float, or dive, or swim, or drown, or ride waves into the water love. She just didn't know when. Until the night she turned fifty-eight. On that night, she sat alone under the moon with her feet at the lip of the ocean. She heard the sea say, hello my love. You are arrived. She heard the sea say, when you were eight, you had to pass through the crucible of child abuse, and you bled. When you were eighteen, you had to pass through the crucible of puberty, and you bled late, since you had been an athlete—you strongest of swimmers. When you were twenty-eight, your daughter died in your belly waters. You bled for her for years, like tears made from blood. When you were thirty-eight, you bled the blood of lust and your son was born. When you were forty-eight, I know, you thought you were dying. You were not dying. You were coming to life. She heard the sea say, tonight you are fifty-eight. Tonight your blood is yours again. You have spent your life giving your human blood to the world, but tonight your blood moves away from human. Your blood circulates again only inside your own body, like a metaphor of all existence. Just as rivers make tributaries all over the world leading to all the oceans, carrying all life, all death, all being, all time. You are the body of water you long for. Come play. The rest of your life is letting the human loose. The rest of your life is joining all being.

And pleasure shuddered her shoulders, and an unnameable cacophonous silence where everyone was expecting a word—no really—there are no words for this—there is no language—came over her in orgasmic unending waves.

You were expecting an ending?

This is not that story. There is no ending but to begin again, as many times as we are offered the chance.

When I write stories, I am conjuring spells, I am shifting meanings, I am undergoing transmogrify. When I hold a rock, and I am a collector of rocks from all over the world, I remember that I am connected to all time and all being and my puny life and body are beautiful because they connect to all other bodies and lives and to the great cosmic expanse. When my body undergoes transmogrify, as it has done my entire life, not just now, for I have been a child, a teenager, an athlete, a worker, a mother, a sister, a wife, a lover, a teacher, a writer, I am shape-shifting into the everything. Maybe take a look at all the bodies you have inhabited and give them their moment of grace. We are here waiting for you to remind you that you are not alone.

As I write this, I am about to be sixty-one. I am on the other side of that place in my story where difficulty seemed the drama. The difficulty now seems like one of many I have endured, and the shape of my story is changing. If you read down into the underworld, you know that I survived that decade of difficulties and pushed into a different body, voice, story. I can look back now and witness what else happened during my menopause decade, and the shift in perspective is everything. In my meno-pause decade, I published possibly the most important books of my life. Five of them. My body shape-shifted along with each book, which now seems incredibly apt; each book required a dif-ferent size and shape. I performed a TED Talk, which has since garnered over 4.5 million views—a story shared over and over again between regular humans. I was of use to some people. This is not nothing, to be useful to others by way of storytelling. It keeps more of us alive. My son just graduated from college, so at least a small minute of motherhood has moved along—whether or not I have been a good mother or a bad mother is not mine to decide, but I do know he feels loved, and that carries worth and weight. My place in the story is thus shifting. Though his life is his and always has been, I had a hand in the story.

As a person who is aging, I have become invisible to my culture in general, but from this vantage point, I can see more clearly that what my culture most wanted from me as I inhabited the space of "woman" for all those years was brutal. Namely, my objectification, my reproductive viability, my sex appeal, my labor, in short, my death, my forfeiting of my own erotic magic, my siphoned agency, my face made-up young, my voice made clean, beautiful, quiet, my storyline shoved into a shape that fits in with and sustains a male social order, or a household, or a nation that keeps me from being fully human. The present tense aging body I now inhabit helps me to help others not lose themselves to the great grand narrative wherein women—meaning anyone stepping into the space of the feminine—serve a patriarchal order. Pssst. Over here. Take this magical side door to fully human, ego distilled, erotic expanse, creative joy. Who gives a shit if I'm invisible? Invisibility is magical, to children. I have become a see-er rather than the one who is endlessly seen. I am on my way to mermaid.

For my sixty-first birthday, I bought myself a wetsuit. To swim in open water. To give myself what I now understand I need. I have shed enough skins to earn a new one.

You might say everything about your body and being has profoundly changed. You might say you are shape-shifting. We are in story space, where everything suddenly becomes possible. Ask yourself what you can give to yourself.

Some of you will find your way back to the natural world elements that cradle all humanity, like my friend Nina who now swims every single day of her life, even as she never swam during any other part of her life. Or like my friend Helga, who has, after knee surgery, taken up rock climbing. Or like my friend Christy, who now runs marathons. Or my friend Camille, who has turned gardening into a life practice. Or my friend Rhonda, who knits and paints on the daily, or my friend Domi, who can not only whistle perfect birdsong but who also had top surgery so they might finally become boy-bodied and touch their joy, or my friend Dena, who sews dolls for refugee children, or all the writers, artists, weavers, beaders, cooks, lawyers, doctors, activists, scientists, and grandmothers I know and stay connected to. I wonder, what is your next becoming?

Others will walk into the forest and remember how trees are the reason we are alive and breathing, so the forest walks and bathing will ease the toil of being human. You can breathe with trees instead of against them. Some of you will find that your voice has been waiting for you all these years. Others will bloom imagination and creativity like flowers shooting out all over your body. Some of you will find help with organic compounds that mimic the body's biology, others may become vegans, or find help from hormone replacement therapies, and the relief you feel—in any form—will be worth it. Look how your radiance takes on a light of your own making. Some of you will find solace in communities through prayer or creativity or meditation. To those of you who choose surgeries, we want you to know that the bowl of your abdomen is like a song reaching up toward the cosmos where other bowls of life are born and die and begin again endlessly. We hold bowls, we pass bowls of life around to one another, we are the bowls. There are stories of bowls and bellies all over the world.

If you find you must eat differently, or sleep differently, or move in the world differently, or grab the hand of someone else who is changing, do it. If you find that you must lay some bodies down in order to continue changing and growing, bodies like rage, or sorrow, or guilt, or shame or fear, or dead love, do it. We honor the parting. We know what weight you carried. Let go. Lift your heart.

Above all, consider creating a ritual any time you need it. Consider conjuring a story every single time you need it. You don't need any special knowledge. You already know how to invent rituals, how to conjure stories.

So let me start this story over again. Not from any ending or beginning, but from the expansive never-endingness of our collective bodies and stories. In this story space where you are reading us, we can be anything.

Congratulations, you fucking spectacular being. You made it. You have come to the threshold of a portal more beautiful than any definition of "beauty" ever shot at you from human culture. You are the sexiest you have ever been. Want to know why? Because your erotic mojo doesn't belong to anyone or anything else. So gush and glow with abandon. Pleasure yourself. Multiply your joy. Share it only when you feel like it. You are released. You don't have to be like anyone else you know. You don't have to compare yourself to anyone or anything else. You are your own universe. You pulsar. You galactic wonder. Your body has gone through the most stunning metamorphoses, beginning with your epic journey exiting the womb, or however you went from breathing water to air. However you came into the world, you are radiant. You may have created life from within your body, or you may have created life by living and loving others in community. Look around you for kin. Not just biological. They may or may not be human or even animate. You may have undergone great transitions, shape-shifting, crucibles, restoryings. You have bled your blood and now that blood is returned to you. Savor the alive. Greet again your own feet, your thighs, the epic poem between your legs, your well-worn gut, your ribs, your heart, your strong shoulders and arms, your neck where voice is held, your head, your face—your astonishing face—and your skin, which carries everything that has ever happened to you like a palimpsest, echoing the cosmos. Let your hair finish its own story; it may be spun into a spider's web that carries the world's stories. Say hello to your new wings, or tail, or scales, or antennae. Your new skin. Your third (or eighth) eye. Your fur, your gills. Your web-making. Your weaving. Your story is fit for fable, myth, fantastic fairy tales, your transmogrify heralds your acceptance into the realm of pure imaginal goo—the much more important than human sphere of butterflies and frogs. You no longer belong to the scriptures and binds of puny humans. Here is your crown, which is made from edible mushrooms. You need no clothing to become in this place. Know that every fold of flesh is loved. Every line or crack or scar is like a poem, like the scar on my mother's leg leading me to my own imagination. Here is your reflection: the entire ocean your eyes, every tree thrusting up from dirt and rooted connection to the cosmos is your hair, your extraordinary heart equal to the aura of the vast night sky. You are all other living beings, all that dies, all that becomes again. You are alive into the everything.

Now sing.

ABOUT THE CONTRIBUTORS

Julia Alvarez left the Dominican Republic for the United States in 1960 at the age of ten. She is the author of six novels, three books of nonfiction, three collections of poetry, and eleven books for children and young adults. Her most recent novel is *The Cemetery of Untold Stories*. *Visitations*, a new collection of poems, will be published in 2026. She has taught and mentored writers in schools and communities across America, and until her retirement in 2016, she was a writer in residence at Middlebury College. Her work has garnered wide recognition, including a Latina Leader Award in Literature from the Congressional Hispanic Caucus Institute, the Hispanic Heritage Award in Literature, being named Woman of the Year by *Latina* magazine, and inclusion in the New York Public Library program "The Hand of the Poet: Original Manuscripts by 100 Masters, from John Donne to Julia Alvarez." *In the Time of the*

Butterflies, with over one million copies in print, was selected by the National Endowment for the Arts for its national Big Read program, and in 2013 President Obama awarded Alvarez the National Medal of Arts in recognition of her extraordinary storytelling. In 2024, she was profiled in "Julia Alvarez: A Life Reimagined" on PBS's *American Masters*. Visit her at www .juliaalvarez.com.

Lan Samantha Chang is the author of *The Family Chao* and three other works of fiction, including *Hunger: A Novella and Stories*. Her writing has been published in *Harper's*, the *Atlantic Monthly*, the *New York Times*, and *The Best American Short Stories*. She has received an Anisfield-Wolf Book Award, a Guggenheim Fellowship, and an Arts and Letters Award in Literature from the American Academy of Arts and Letters. She lives with her family in Iowa City, Iowa, where she directs the Iowa Writers' Workshop.

Nana-Ama Danquah is an author, editor, freelance journalist, ghostwriter, public speaker, actress, and teacher. Her groundbreaking memoir, *Willow Weep for Me: A Black Woman's Journey Through Depression* was hailed by the *Washington Post* as "a vividly textured flower of a memoir, one of the finest to come along in years." A native of Ghana, Ms. Danquah is editor of four anthologies: *Becoming American: Personal Essays by First Generation Immigrant Women*; *Shaking the Tree: New Fiction and Memoir by Black Women*; *The Black Body*; and *Accra Noir*, as part of Akashic's popular noir series. Ms. Danquah earned a Master of Fine Arts degree in Creative Writing and Literature from Bennington College. Her writing has been featured in magazines, newspapers, and literary journals. Her essays and poems have been heavily anthologized and used in high school and university textbooks. As a ghostwriter, Ms. Danquah has written numerous *New York Times* bestsellers for clients. From 2012 to 2016, she was the International Speechwriter for H.E. John Dramani Mahama, the President of Ghana. In that capacity, she wrote four United Nations General Assembly speeches and various addresses and keynotes delivered by President Mahama at high-level conferences, meetings, and panels.

Monica Drake is the author of the novels *Clown Girl* and *The Stud Book*, as well as the linked story collection, *The Folly of Loving Life*. Her essays and short fiction have appeared in the *New York Times'* "Modern Love," the *Paris Review*, the *Sun*, *Oregon Humanities Magazine*, *Longreads*, and other venues.

Gina Frangello's fifth book, the memoir *Blow Your House Down: A Story of Family, Feminism, and Treason* (Counterpoint), was selected as a *New York Times* Editor's Choice, received starred reviews in *Publishers Weekly*, *Library Journal*, and *BookPage*, and was included on numerous "Best of 2021" lists including at *Lithub*, *BookPage*, and *The Chicago Review of Books*. Her sixth book, *Elena Ferrante: The Neapolitan Novels*, was released as part of IG Publishing's "Bookmarked" series in July 2024. Gina is also the author of four books of fiction, most recently *A Life in Men* and *Every Kind of Wanting*, and her debut novel and short story collection, *My Sister's Continent* and *Slut Lullabies*, are being reissued by Northwestern University Press in fall 2026. Gina has also worked as an editor for more than a quarter century, having founded both the independent press

Other Voices Books and the fiction section of The Nervous Breakdown, as well as serving as the Sunday editor for *The Rumpus*, the faculty editor for both *TriQuarterly Online* and the *Coachella Review*, and the Creative Nonfiction Editor for the *Los Angeles Review of Books*. Gina obtained her PhD in English/Creative Writing from the University of Illinois Chicago, with a specialization in Gender Theory. She is on the low residency MFA faculty at the University of Nevada-Reno/Tahoe and runs Circe Consulting, a full-service company for writers, with the writer Emily Rapp Black.

Roxane Gay is the author of several bestselling books and has an imprint, Roxane Gay Books, at Grove Atlantic.

Reyna Grande was born in Guerrero, Mexico, and is the author of the bestselling memoirs *The Distance Between Us* and *A Dream Called Home*, as well as the novels *Across a Hundred Mountains*, *Dancing with Butterflies*, and *A Ballad of Love and Glory*, a novel set during the US invasion of Mexico in the 1840s. She is the co-editor of an anthology by and about undocumented Americans called *Somewhere We Are Human: Authentic Voices on Migration, Survival and New Beginnings*. Her books have been adopted as the common read selection by schools, colleges, and cities nationwide. Reyna has received several awards, including an American Book Award, the El Premio Aztlán Literary Award, and a Writers for Writers Award from Poets & Writers. Her two forthcoming projects are a collection of personal essays and an anthology on Sandra Cisneros. Visit her at reynagrande.com.

Pam Houston is the author of the short story collection *Cowboys Are My Weakness*, the memoir *Deep Creek: Finding*

Hope in the High Country, and six other books of fiction and nonfiction. Her books have won multiple Western States, Mountains and Plains and Colorado Book Awards and her stories have appeared in *The Best American Short Stories*, the *O Henry Prize Anthology*, and *The Best American Short Stories of the Century*. She teaches creative writing at the Institute of American Indian Arts and UC Davis and is cofounder and creative director of the literary nonprofit Writing by Writers and fiction editor at the environmental arts journal Terrain.org. She lives on a homestead at nine thousand feet near the headwaters of the Rio Grande. Her book *Without Exception: Reclaiming Abortion, Personhood and Freedom* was published by Torrey House Press in September.

Nguyễn Phan Quế Mai is an award-winning writer in both Vietnamese and English languages. She is the author of thirteen books of poetry, nonfiction, and fiction, most recently the global bestselling novels *The Mountains Sing* and *Dust Child*. Her writing has received the PEN Oakland/Josephine Miles Literary Award, the International Book Award, the BookBrowse Best Debut Award, the Lannan Literary Fellowship in Fiction as well as runner-up for the Dayton Literary Peace Prize—the first and only annual US literary award recognizing the power of the written word to promote peace. Quế Mai's writing has been translated into more than twenty-five languages. She was named by Forbes Việt Nam as one of twenty inspiring women of 2021 and recently by the Research House of Asia as one of the Top 10 Female Novelists Shaping the Literary Scene in Southeast Asia. For more information: nguyenphanquemai.com.

Joey Soloway is a trans philosopher and public intellectual. As a filmmaker they created *Transparent, Afternoon Delight*, and *I Love Dick*. They are currently completing the South Commons Experiment, a documentary about their childhood experience growing up in a "utopian" community on the South Side of Chicago. Joey wrote the books *She Wants It* and *Tiny Ladies in Shiny Pants*, as well as various comedic essays you can find scattered throughout the internet. They're available to come to your institution and do their one-person show *The Three Thousand Year Old Them*.

Darcey Steinke is the author of the forthcoming book *This Is the Door: The Body, Pain and Faith*. She has published both novels and memoirs and she often writes about art. Her books have been translated into ten languages, and her writing has appeared among other places in the *New York Times Magazine*, the *New Yorker*, the *Paris Review*, *Vogue*, *Spin Magazine*, and the *Guardian*. Her web story "Blindspot" was a part of the 2000 Whitney Biennial and she was short-listed last year for the French Arles Author Prize. Darcey has taught at The New School, Columbia, Princeton, and the American University of Paris.

Cheryl Strayed is the author of the #1 *New York Times* bestseller *Wild: From Lost to Found on the Pacific Crest Trail*, which was made into an Oscar-nominated film. Her bestselling collection of Dear Sugar columns, *Tiny Beautiful Things*, was adapted for a Hulu television show and as a play that continues to be staged in theaters nationwide. Strayed's other books are the critically acclaimed novel *Torch* and the bestselling collection *Brave Enough*. Her writing has been published in *The Best American Essays*, the *New York Times*, the *Washington Post Magazine*, *Vogue*, and elsewhere.

Lidia Yuknavitch is the bestselling author of the memoirs *Reading the Waves* and *The Chronology of Water*, the novels *Thrust*, *The Book of Joan*, *The Small Backs of Children*, and *Dora: A Headcase*, and is the winner of the Oregon Book Award. Her TED Talk, "On the Beauty of Being a Misfit," has over four million views. She founded the arts organization Corporeal Writing in Portland, Oregon. Lidia has a PhD in literature from the University of Oregon. She is a very good swimmer and hopes to finish evolving back into a water creature sooner than later.

PERMISSIONS